Barb Smith

CONCEPTS IN

MEDICAL

RADIOGRAPHIC

IMAGING:

INSTRUCTOR'S GUIDE

CONCEPTS IN
MEDICAL
RADIOGRAPHIC
IMAGING:
INSTRUCTOR'S GUIDE

Marianne Tortorici, Ed.D., RT(R)
Professor
University of Nevada, Las Vegas

Hiram M. Hunt, Ed.D., RRPT
Professor (Retired)
University of Nevada, Las Vegas

W. B. SAUNDERS CO.
HARCOURT BRACE JOVANOVICH, INC.
PHILADELPHIA LONDON TORONTO MONTREAL SYDNEY TOKYO

W. B. Saunders Company
Harcourt Brace Jovanovich, Inc.

The Curtis Center
Independence Square West
Philadelphia, Pennsylvania 19106

Editor: Lisa A. Biello

Designer: Paul Fry

Production Manager: Linda R. Garber

Illustration Specialist: Peg Shaw

Concepts in Medical Radiographic Imaging: Instructor's Guide   ISBN   0-7216-3118-5

Printed in the United States of America.

Last digit is the print number: 9   8   7   6   5   4   3   2   1

We wish to thank our students at the University of Nevada, Las Vegas, for their comments concerning the original laboratory experiments from which this manual was developed.

PREFACE

As educators for a combined 40 years, we have learned that "Murphy's Law" always seems to apply to laboratory experiments. No matter how many times we have performed an experiment, there always seems to be one student who finds an innovative way of achieving "unusual" results. Such results often frustrate the learner and educator alike. Therefore, this guide is written to share our experiences with other educators in an attempt to limit those "unusual" results and frustrating experiences.

All experiments in the laboratory manual have been conducted for several years at the University of Nevada, Las Vegas. Many of the laboratory experiments were published by us in a previous manual and used at several radiography schools. The suggestions and comments we received from our own students and from educators at other schools have enabled us to polish the laboratory experiments. The suggestions herein are intended to help educators adapt these laboratory experiments to their classroom situations.

Because conditions vary from one school to another, some suggestions found in this guide may work well in your program while others may not. It should be noted that because the specific data recorded by a particular experimenter, e.g., voltage measurements, cannot be known to the authors, suggestions for answers to the data and conclusion sections in this guide are based upon a general summarization of the normally expected results. The instructor may wish to request that the researchers be more specific in their conclusions to meet the needs of the respective schools.

CONTENTS

SECTION I

CIRCUITRY AND EQUIPMENT EXPERIMENTS

1 Magnetism 1

2 Electrical Symbols and Diagrams 4

3 Electromagnetism 7

4 Resistors 10

5 Multitesters 12

6 Production of Electricity 16

7 Ohm's Law 19

8 Series Circuits 21

9 Parallel Circuits 24

10 Step Up and Step Down Transformers 26

11 Transformer Power and Efficiency 28

12 Rectification 30

13 Timer Tests 32

14 Density and Exposure Measuring Devices 35

15 Automatic Timers 38

16 Focal Spot Size 40

17 Heel Effect 42

18   Kilovoltage Compensation 44

19   Kilovoltage Check 46

20   Half-Value Layer 48

21   Effect of Kilovoltage on Contrast 49

22   Milliampere Check 51

23   Law of Reciprocity 54

24   Effect of Milliampere-Seconds on Density 57

25   Tomography: Fulcrum Level 59

26   Tomography: Effect of Exposure Angle on Thickness of
     Objective Plane 61

SECTION II

FILM PROCESSING AND PHOTOGRAPHIC TECHNIQUES EXPERIMENTS

27   Processing Area Design 63

28   Processing Area Quality Control 65

29   Processor Parts and Function 67

30   Processor Inspection 70

31   Subtraction 73

32   Stereoradiography 75

33   Film Duplication 77

34   Sensitometry 79

35   Silver Recovery 81

SECTION III

FACTORS AFFECTING FILM QUALITY EXPERIMENTS

36   Intensifying Light Screen Emission 83

37   Intensifying Screen Resolution 85

38   Intensifying Screen Contact 87

39 Grid Lines 89

40 Grid Cutoff 91

41 Beam Restrictors: X-ray Beam and Light Accuracy 93

42 Effect of Distortion on Radiographic Quality 95

43 Effect of Magnification on Radiographic Quality 97

44 Effect of Motion on Radiographic Quality 100

45 Inverse Square Law 102

46 Added Filtration 104

47 Reject Film Analysis 106

HOW TO BUILD A CIRCUIT BOARD

The circuit boards listed for the electrical laboratories are easily and inexpensively constructed by anyone with some skill and basic tools. The following is a pictorial step-by-step process for constructing a circuit board.

Step 1: Parts

Figure 1 demonstrates all the parts needed to build the circuit board. These items can be purchased in any hardware or electrical store, e.g., Radio Shack. When purchasing these items, the following need be considered:

1. Battery holds are available in many sizes. The laboratories in this manual allow the experimenter to use either size "C" or "D" batteries. Thus, the instructor should purchase battery holders to match the specific size battery that will be used for the experiments. The holders the authors use are made to hold two batteries preconnected in series.

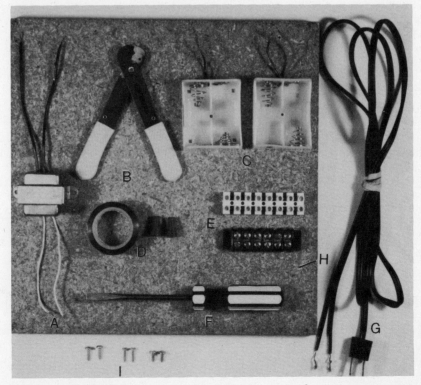

Figure 1. Items needed to build a circuit board: A. step-down transformer, B. wire stripper and cutter, C. battery holders, D. electrical tape or wire connectors, E. terminal strip, F. flat head screwdriver, G. electrical extension cord, H. wooden board, and I. screws.

2. It is strongly recommended that transformers NO GREATER than a 1:24 ratio be purchased.

3. There are several types of terminal strips available. Two are illustrated in Figure 1. The authors originally used the type with screws on top (see the bottom item E in Figure 1). However, by the end of the first semester of work, the ends of the resistors and other electrical components broke from constantly bending the ends to fit under the screw. It was decided to replace the terminal with one that allows the ends of electrical components to be inserted in a hollow connector underneath the screw (see the top item E in Figure 1). This type of terminal has reduced the number of ancillary electrical items needing replacement.

4. The wires may be spliced with electrical tape or wire connectors. If wire connectors are used, the size should match the specific gauge wire being used.

Step 2: Connecting the Transformer to the Electrical Cord

Cut off the female end of the electrical extension cord so that only the male end (the plug that enters a wall socket) remains. Use the wire cutters to strip the ends of each wire. Use electrical tape or wire connectors (Fig. 2) to connect the ends of the electrical cord to the side of the step-down transformer with the HIGHEST NUMBER OF TURNS.

The transformer or box the transformer came in usually identifies the transformer ratio. Some transformers have the same number of wires on the primary and secondary sides; most have three wires on one side (the middle wire is a ground AND IS CONNECTED TO A FREE TERMINAL SCREW—DO NOT CONNECT THE GROUND TO THE CIRCUIT WHEN PERFORMING EXPERIMENTS) and two wires on the other side. In cases where there are two wires on one side and three on the other, the side with three wires represents the secondary side of the transformer. In cases were transformers have the same number of wires, the primary and secondary sides should be labeled on the transformer.

If a step-down transformer having a 24:1 ratio is used, the primary side (the side with two wires) must be connected to the electrical cord because it has the highest number of turns. The reverse is true if the transformer is a step-up transformer (1:24). FAILURE TO CONNECT THE CORRECT SIDE TO MAKE THE TRANSFORMER A STEP-DOWN TRANSFORMER MAY RESULT IN INCREASING THE 110 VOLTS TO THOUSANDS OF VOLTS.

Step 3: Positioning of Components

Position the transformer, battery holder, and terminal on the wooden board so both the battery wires and transformer wires can easily reach the terminal. Leave enough space to attach resistors, diodes, etc., for laboratory work.

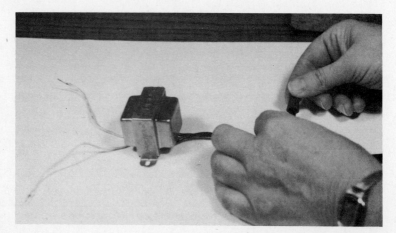

Figure 2. Splice the electrical cord to the transformer.

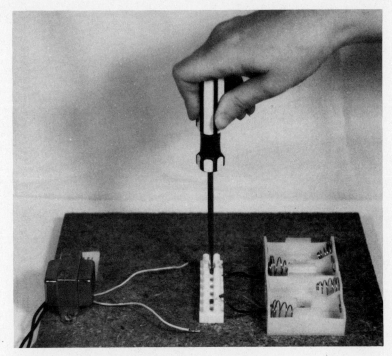

Figure 3. Secure the items to the wooden board.

Step 4: Securing the Components

After you are satisfied with the location of the items, use the screws to secure them to the wooden board (Fig. 3). Most transformers come with a diagram of the ratio. It is recommended that the diagram be attached to the wooden board near the transformer, especially for transformers that are not labeled with a ratio.

MAGNETISM

Care should be taken not to store magnetic compasses next to magnets; a magnet may cause the compass to become inoperable. If the north-seeking pole of the compass needle is no longer pointing north, as it should, the compass needle may be "realigned" with the bar magnet. To "realign" a compass, simply place the compass on top of the magnet and rapidly move the compass longitudinally over the magnet. If this does not realign the compass, the magnet may be too weak or change the location of the poles, e.g., reverse the magnet.

EQUIPMENT

Because magnetic field direction is important, it is suggested that bar magnets which have the north and south poles labeled be employed. One popular manufacturer of this type of magnet is Sargent-Welch Scientific Co., 1617 E. Ball Road, P. O. Box 4038, Anaheim, CA 92803.

Iron filings are easily obtained from any industry that generates iron filings as scrap (avoid oily or greasy filings). Another possible source is a physics, metallurgy or engineering department within your school. If these sources are unavailable, it is possible to make your own filings by simply filing some soft iron. It is recommended that the filings be stored, as they are reusable. They can be demagnetized by shaking them in a bottle.

Ferromagnetic and nonferromagnetic materials are readily available at any company which has scrap metal or hardware stores. Other sources are physics or engineering departments, etc., which may be on your campus. It is recommended that a number be stamped on each of the metals for easy identification.

MATERIAL

Due to the fact some support is necessary to hold the iron filings, a rather rigid cardboard should be used. A regular cardboard folder used for filing office papers is more than adequate. Regular tablet paper should not be used as a support.

E X P E R I M E N T 1

V I S U A L O B S E R V A T I O N

The diagram of the compass and magnet should demonstrate flux lines that travel from the north to the south. The diagram with iron filings cannot demonstrate direction, but will display the lines surrounding the magnet. The lines should be more concentrated at the poles than at the sides.

C O N C L U S I O N

The compass demonstrated that flux lines existed and travelled from the north to south pole. The iron filings displayed the magnetic flux lines surrounding the magnet. The lines were more concentrated at the poles.

E X P E R I M E N T 2

V I S U A L O B S E R V A T I O N

The diagram with the like poles should show the iron filings moving away from each other. The diagram with unlike poles displays the iron filings "connecting" or attracting each other.

C O N C L U S I O N

Like poles repel each other and unlike poles attract each other.

E X P E R I M E N T 3

V I S U A L O B S E R V A T I O N

The experimenter should identify which metals were attracted by the magnet. The experimenter should not attempt to identify the metal by name, e.g., aluminum.

C O N C L U S I O N

The researcher should identify, by number, the metals which were ferromagnetic and nonferromagnetic. Since these metals are unknown to the researcher, the data does not support the ability of the experimenter to list the metal by name.

ANSWERS TO QUESTIONS

1. Define magnetism.

Magnetism may be defined as a class of physical phenomena that includes the attraction for iron exhibited by lodestone and other magnetized materials.

2. State the three laws of magnetism.

There are three fundamental laws of magnetism: (1) every magnet has two poles, (2) like poles repel each other, unlike poles attract each other and (3) the force of attraction or repulsion between two magnetic poles is directly proportional to the strength of the poles and indirectly proportional to the square of the distance between them.

3. List two characteristics of magnetic flux lines.

One characteristic of flux lines is the manner in which they travel. Flux lines travel parallel to each other. On the exterior aspect of the magnet, the flux lines travel from the north pole of the magnet to the magnetic south pole. Within the magnet, flux line flow is from the south pole to the north pole. A second characteristic of magnetic flux is that flux lines flowing in the same direction repel while those moving in the opposite direction attract. The last characteristic of flux lines is that flux lines are distorted when a magnetic material is placed in the field and are unaffected when a nonmagnetic material is positioned in the flux path.

4. List three types of materials that exhibit magnetic properties.

Three types of magnetic materials are paramagnetic, diamagnetic and ferromagnetic.

5. What are the characteristics of a ferromagnetic material?

Ferromagnetic material is easily magnetized. The material takes on the opposite polarity of the magnetic pole magnetizing it. These materials make the strongest magnets.

6. How can a magnetic field be detected?

A magnetic field may be detected by a compass or iron filings.

LABORATORY

2

ELECTRICAL
SYMBOLS AND
DIAGRAMS

This laboratory is best performed with the students divided into small groups. It is designed to introduce the researcher to electrical symbols, to teach the experimenter how to read circuit diagrams and to enable the researcher to properly construct a circuit. Because a large percentage of the succeeding laboratories utilize this basic information, it is recommended that all students demonstrate competency before being permitted to perform additional laboratory experiments. Permitting students who did not demonstrate competency to continue often results in the researcher becoming frustrated because he/she is unable to perform the succeeding experiments.

One useful method of insuring that every student understands this laboratory is to limit class size to a maximum of fifteen. Another helpful way to facilitate learning is to employ, as assistants, former students who have already successfully completed the course or any other individual who is competent in basic electricity. Also, these individuals may be employed as tutors after the laboratory experience. A third method is to lecture on the topic before actually performing the experiments.

Experiment number 1 should be performed first. The sequence of experiments number 2 and 3 is irrelevant. If the quantity of equipment available is limited, it is recommended that some groups perform experiment number 2 while others perform experiment number 3.

EQUIPMENT

The equipment employed in this laboratory is inexpensive and readily available through any electrical store. For information on how to build your own circuit board, refer to the "How to Build a Circuit Board" section of the Introduction to this instructor's guide.

EXPERIMENT 1

CONCLUSION

There are electrical symbols which may be used to identify electrical components. Some symbols greatly resemble the component while others have little similarity to the item.

EXPERIMENT 2

CIRCUIT CONSTRUCTION

It is recommended that each group member be assigned a specific task when performing this experiment. Assignable tasks include reading the diagram and giving instructions to others, selecting the electrical components and placing the electrical components in the circuit.

Another method to consider when performing this experiment is to have the researcher rotate his/her tasks from circuit A to circuit B, etc. This provides a means for the researcher to experience all aspects of the experiment.

CONCLUSION

By interpreting electrical symbols, it is possible to construct an electrical circuit.

EXPERIMENT 3

PROCEDURE

The instructor should set up and label ("1" and "2" or "A" and "B") the example circuits. The circuits should be simple. It is recommended that they be constructed differently than those in experiment number 2. Care should be taken to avoid keeping the circuits connected for too long, which results in heating up of the electrical components or batteries.

DATA

The experimenter must draw an electrical diagram which accurately reflects the circuit constructed by the instructor.

CONCLUSION

It is possible to use electrical symbols to diagram a circuit.

ANSWERS TO QUESTIONS

1. Draw and label the electrical symbols for the following items: battery, resistor, semiconductor diode, transformer and voltmeter.

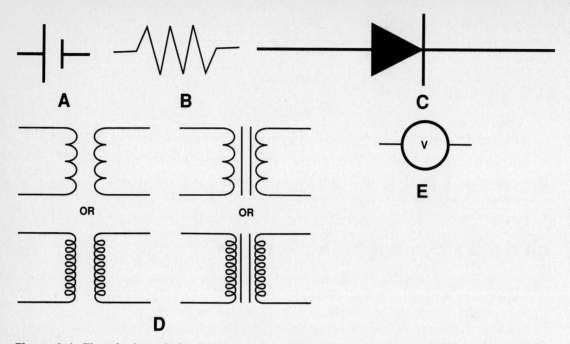

Figure 2–1. Electrical symbols. A, battery, B, resistor, C, semiconductor diode, D, traformer, and E, voltmeter.

Figure 2–1 shows the symbols for question number 1.

2. Draw a circuit which has the following characteristics: four batteries in series, two resistors in parallel.

Figure 2–2 represents the circuit for question number 2.

3. In your own words, describe the electrical circuit diagramed in Figure 2–5 (from the Laboratory Manual) below:

Figure 2–5 is a transformer connected to 2 resistors in series.

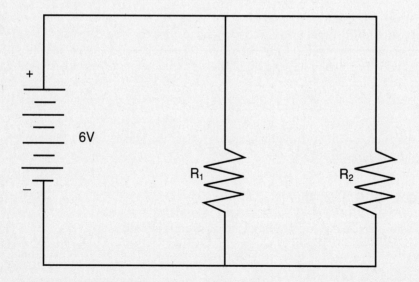

Figure 2–2. Diagram for question number 2.

3

ELECTRO-MAGNETISM

Prior to performing this laboratory, the researcher needs to have some knowledge of how to construct a simple circuit from a diagram. Thus, it is recommended that the instructor provide the researcher some guidance in this area (see electrical symbols and diagrams laboratory). The experimenter should also be directed as to how to use the cross section conductor symbols. The cross section symbol representing current moving away from the experiment (moving "into" this page) is $\otimes$. The symbol O is used to represent current flow toward the researcher (moving "up" from this page).

It does not matter which experiment, number 1 or number 2, is performed first. However, it is recommended that the experimenter perform both experiments.

The electrical materials for this laboratory may be obtained inexpensively at any electrical or hardware store. The instructor is referred to the "How to build a circuit board" section in the introduction portion of this guide.

The compass should be checked for accuracy prior to beginning the experiment. If the compass needle is not pointing in the proper direction (the earth's north pole), it may need to be realigned. The compass may be realigned by placing it on a magnet and moving it rapidly over the magnet from one end (pole) of the magnet to the other until the north pole of the compass needle points north. If this does not realign the compass, the magnet may be too weak or change the location of the poles, e.g., reverse the magnet.

EXPERIMENT 1

PROCEDURE

Use enough batteries to have a detectable magnetic flow (this laboratory recommends a minimum of 4). Avoid using a conductor with a high resistance. This will hinder the flow of electricity.

The length of the conductor should be long enough to hold it vertical so a compass can be moved around the conductor freely. Care should be taken not to use a conductor which is too long, as length increases resistance.

This experiment is best performed with one person holding about 5 inches of the conductor in a vertical position; a second person may then rotate the compass 360° around the conductor (make sure the compass is at a 90° angle to the conductor). The person rotating the compass should read the direction of the needle approximately every 60° to a third person who records the reading.

VISUAL OBSERVATION

The experimenter may try to read the compass relative to north, south, east or west. The magnetic field of the conductor is stronger than the earth's magnetic field and overrides the compass' ability to point to the earth's north pole. Therefore, the experimenter must record the compass needle relative to the position of the needle.

CONCLUSION

The direction of the magnetic field which accompanies the flow of an electric current through a single wire conductor is circular and perpendicular to the path of the current flow through the conductor.

EXPERIMENT 2

PROCEDURE

A simple coiled wire can be made by wrapping a low resistant conductor around a cardboard tube, e.g., the cardboard found inside of tissue paper or paper towel. Sometimes the length of the wire creates a large resistance and the magnetic field of the conductor is too weak to be detected. To increase the magnetic field in this case, insert several 12 or 16 penny common nails inside the coil. Be aware that nails tend to retain the magnetism. Thus, if the nails are used from one laboratory to another, always be sure they are in an unmagnetized state prior to performing the experiment.

VISUAL OBSERVATION

As with experiment number 1, the experimenter may try to read the compass relative to north, south, east or west. The magnetic field of the conductor is stronger than the earth's magnetic field. Therefore, the experimenter must record the needle of the compass relative to the position of the needle.

CONCLUSION

The magnetic field produced by a flow of electrons through a coil is a composite of the magnetic fields produced by the current flowing in the individual increments (turns) of the coil such that the coiled wire demonstrates a north and south pole.

ANSWERS TO QUESTIONS

1. Define "electromagnetism."

Electromagnetism is that branch of physics which deals with the physical relations between electricity and magnetism.

2. In what direction do electrons flow in a circuit?

Electrons flow from the negative pole of a voltaic cell through the circuit to the positive pole.

3. What is the direction of the magnetic field relative to the path of the electrical current which generates it?

The direction of the magnetic field which accompanies the flow of an electric current through a conductor is circular and perpendicular to the path of the current flow through the conductor.

4. What is the advantage of using a coiled wire vs. a single straight wire for a conductor when trying to produce an electromagnetic field?

The advantage of using a coil vs. a straight wire to produce a magnetic field is that the magnetic field produced by doing so is stronger for the same amount of current.

4

RESISTORS

Many of the succeeding laboratories require the use of resistors. Thus, mastery of this laboratory is essential to properly complete other laboratories. Permitting researchers who do not demonstrate competency to continue often results in the researcher becoming frustrated because he/she is unable to perform the succeeding experiments.

One useful method of ensuring that every individual understands this laboratory is to limit class size to a maximum of fifteen. Another helpful way to facilitate learning is to employ, as assistants, former students who have already successfully completed the course or any other individual who is competent in basic electricity. Also, these individuals may be employed as tutors after the laboratory experience. A third method is to lecture on the topic before actually performing the experiments.

PROCEDURE

Sometimes the color codes of resistors are difficult to read, e.g., violet may appear as a dark brown. Also, some researchers may be color blind. Thus, it is recommended that the instructor visually review all resistors with each experimenter to ensure he/she is able to read the colors properly.

Resistors are available in a wide range of values. The researcher should select a variety of different values. It is recommended that the instructor encourage the experimenter to use scientific notation (see appendix B of the Student Manual) for resistors having a resistance in the hundreds of thousands of ohms.

DATA

The data depend upon the resistors selected. The instructor may wish to double check the researcher's mathematics by measuring the resistor with an ohmmeter.

CONCLUSION

The resistance and accuracy (tolerance) of a resistor can be determined by reading the color code. Some resistors are more accurate than others.

ANSWERS TO QUESTIONS

1. Fill in the blanks for the following resistor code chart.

| Resistor Number | Band number | | | | Numerical Value of Code | Tolerance | Ohm Range |
	1	2	3	4			
1	Orange	Black	Orange	None	30,000	± 20%	24,000-36,000
2	Orange	Black	Silver	Silver	0.3	± 10%	0.27-0.33
3	Violet	Green	Gold	Gold	7.5	± 5%	7.125-7.875
4	Brown	Violet	Yellow	Silver	170,000	± 10%	153,000-187,000
5	Black	Orange	Black	None	3	± 20%	2.4-3.6

2. What determines the value in ohms of a resistor.

The type of resistance material and the cross-sectional area and length of the resistance material in its case determine the resistance value of the resistor in ohms.

3. Identify one reason for using an electrical resistor?

Resistors are useful when inserted in an electrical circuit to reduce current flow that might damage a circuit component.

5

MULTITESTERS

Prior to performing this laboratory, the researcher should have tested competent in the electrical symbols and diagrams and resistor laboratories.

Many of the succeeding laboratories require the use of a multitester. Thus, mastery of this laboratory is essential to properly complete other laboratories. Permitting researchers who do not demonstrate competency to continue often results in the researcher becoming frustrated because he/she is unable to perform the succeeding experiments.

One useful method of ensuring that every individual understands this laboratory is to limit class size to a maximum of fifteen. Another helpful way to facilitate learning is to employ, as assistants, former students who have already successfully completed the course or any other individual who is competent in basic electricity. Also, these individuals may be employed as tutors after the laboratory experience. A third method is to lecture on the topic before actually performing the experiments.

EQUIPMENT

If a multitester which has a scale versus a digital readout is used, it is suggested that a transparency or slide of the scale and face of the meter (showing probe and dial connections) be made. The transparency or slide may be projected on a movie screen and used to demonstrate to experimenters the proper probe connections, dial settings and method of reading the scale (use a pencil or other object to show needle placement on the scale).

The expense of materials and equipment in this laboratory may be kept at a minimum. The greatest expense is the multitester. It is recommended that the instructor check several commercial sources before purchasing a multitester. Prior to purchasing a multitester, the instructor should determine whether a digital readout or a numerical scale is most convenient. To be able to utilize the meter for other laboratories in the manual, the meter should have the capacity to read AC voltage, DC voltage, ohms, and DC milliamperage. One experiment does require an AC current meter. A second separate meter may be required to read AC milliampere. The following are minimal ranges for the various units:

0-120 AC volts

0-10 DC volts

0-15,000 ohms

0-1,000 DC milliamperes

0-1,000 AC milliamperes

Check the instruction sheet of the multitester prior to purchase. You may need to buy batteries to operate the meter.

It is possible for the batteries of the battery operated multitester to become weak with use or age; check to make sure the batteries are still strong before using the multitester. Care should also be taken to turn off the meters after using them to extend the life of the batteries.

Sometimes the ends of the probes loosen or become unscrewed with use. Check the ends to insure that they are tight prior to using the multitester.

For information on how to build your own circuit board, refer to the "How to Build a Circuit Board" section of this guide.

DATA FOR EXPERIMENTS 1, 2 AND 3

The specific readings depend upon the resistance of the circuit.

EXPERIMENT 1

PROCEDURE

Make sure the researchers have read the multitester's instructions prior to performing this experiment. Due to the fact that the meter may be damaged if its probes are placed in the circuit improperly, it is recommended that the instructor quiz the experimenters verbally concerning where the probes will be placed in the circuit. It is advisable to stress that voltage is measured by placing the probes of the meter in parallel with the load and milliamperage is measured by placing the probes of the meter in series with the load. The greatest problem tends to be researchers who forget to open the circuit to measure resistance.

CONCLUSION

A multitester may be employed to measure the voltage of a circuit. The voltage of a circuit is measured by placing the multitester in parallel with the load. This experiment is intended to allow the researcher to use multitesters, thus, any reference to the relationship of voltage in a series circuit is inappropriate. There is a specific laboratory, Series circuits, that deals with this concept.

EXPERIMENT 2

CONCLUSION

A multitester may be employed to measure the current of a circuit. The current of a circuit is measured by placing the multitester in series with the load. This experiment is intended to allow the researcher to use multitesters, thus, any reference to the relationship of current in a series circuit is inappropriate. There is a specific laboratory, Series circuits, that deals with this concept.

EXPERIMENT 3

PROCEDURE

To stabilize the resistor during measurement, it may be connected to an open terminal on the circuit board. If the resistor is not connected to the circuit board, a need exists to make sure the experimenter does not touch the probes of the meter while measuring the resistance. Doing so will also measure the resistance of the human body. Thus, the researcher may wish to place the resistor on a flat surface and touch the probes to the resistor.

CONCLUSION

A multitester may be employed to measure the resistance of a resistor. The resistance of a resistor is determined by measuring the resistor with the multitester in an open circuit.

ANSWERS TO QUESTIONS

1. Indicate by drawing the correct symbol in Figure 5–4 of the Laboratory Manual where the probes for multitester are placed to measure the voltage of r_2.

   Refer to Figure 5–1 for the answer to question number 1.

2. Indicate by drawing the correct symbol in Figure 5–5 of the Laboratory Manual where the probes of a multitester are placed to correctly measure the amperes of r_1.

   Refer to Figure 5–2 for the answer to question number 2.

3. Why isn't resistance measured in a closed circuit?

   Resistance should not be measured in a closed circuit because the meter may be damaged or destroyed if an electric current is flowing through the resistor when its resistance is being measured.

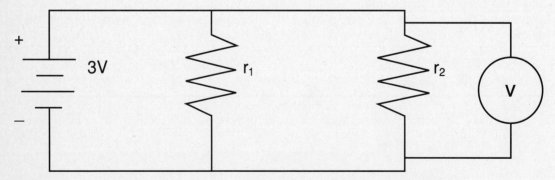

Figure 5–1. Location of the probes for a voltmeter measuring the voltage over r_2.

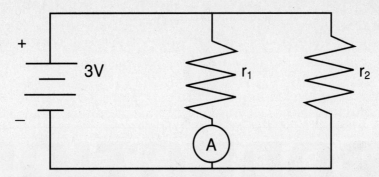

Figure 5–2. Location of the probes for a milliammeter measuring the current over r_1.

6

PRODUCTION

OF

ELECTRICITY

The introduction section of the laboratory identifies 3 ways to produce electricity and 4 factors affecting the current strength. This laboratory demonstrates 2 of the 3 ways to produce electricity. They are moving a magnet through a stationary coil and moving a coil over a stationary magnet. Also, 2 of the 4 factors affecting current strength are illustrated in the laboratory. The factors demonstrated are number of turns in the coil and the speed with which the conductor is "cut" by the magnetic field. If the instructor has access to 2 different strength magnets, he/she may wish to demonstrate the affect of varying strength on the quantity of the current.

It does not matter which experiment is performed first. However, since all 3 experiments serve to explain the concept of the production of electricity, all should be performed.

EQUIPMENT

The equipment in this laboratory is inexpensive. The galvanometer or milliammeter represents the greatest expense. Before purchasing a galvanometer, it is recommended that the instructor locate one that indicates the quantity of current (in mA) and is able to show direction. If a galvanometer which only shows direction can be located, it should be used for experiments number 1 and 2. However, a mA meter for measuring DC amperes must be employed for experiment number 3.

The magnet should be either a bar or cylinder. This facilitates the independent movement of the magnet and coil wire.

The 2 sets of coiled wires must be of the same material and thickness. Also, the wire must be long enough to wrap around a cardboard (the cardboard found inside of tissue paper or paper towel serves as an excellent holder) at least 15 times for the single layer and 45 times for the 3 layered coil. The opening of the coil must be large enough to allow the magnet to pass freely through it.

After the coil is wrapped around a cardboard, the length of the coil should not be greater than 1/3 the length of the magnet. If the coil is too long, it makes it difficult to move the magnet and conductor independently.

E X P E R I M E N T   1

P R O C E D U R E

It is suggested that one person hold the coiled wire and a second person move the magnet. The magnet must move in one direction only. Moving the magnet back and forth within the coil generates alternating current.

If the galvanometer needle does not move, check to see that the wire is connected to the meter. If the galvanometer needle still does not move, increase the number of turns of the coil or the strength of the magnet.

D A T A

The researcher should be able to identify the direction the needle moved relative to the polarity of the magnet. Many galvanometers identify direction by using "+" and "-" symbols.

C O N C L U S I O N

When the north end of the magnet entered the coil first, current moved toward the negative end of the galvanometer. As the south end of the magnet entered the coil, the current flowed in the opposite direction as when the north pole was placed in the coil first.

An electric current can be generated by moving a magnet over a stationary conductor.

E X P E R I M E N T   2

P R O C E D U R E

It is suggested that one person hold the magnet and a second person move the conductor. The conductor must move in one direction only. Moving the conductor back and forth over the magnet generates alternating current.

If the galvanometer needle does not move, check to see that the wire is connected to the meter. If the galvanometer needle still does not move, increase the number of turns of the coil or the strength of the magnet.

D A T A

The researcher should be able to identify the direction the needle moved relative to the polarity of the magnet. Many galvanometers identify direction by using "+" and "-" symbols.

CONCLUSION

When the coil moved over the magnet from north to south, current moved toward the negative end of the galvanometer. As the conductor moved over the magnet south to north, the current flowed in the opposite direction as when the coil moved over the magnet north to south.

An electric current can be generated by moving a conductor over a stationary magnet.

EXPERIMENT 3

PROCEDURE

This experiment requires that the amperage be measured. Consequently, the researcher must use a galvanometer or milliammeter which can measure the quantity of the current.

The introduction mentions speed of the conductor, yet this experiment is written to move the magnet. The effect is identical. If the instructor wishes, he/she may elect to have the researcher move the conductor for consistency. However, experience of the author has demonstrated that it is easier to move the magnet in a rapid fashion rather than the coil.

DATA

The data should demonstrate an increase in the current as the speed of the magnet and the number of turns increase.

CONCLUSION

The strength of the current increases as the speed of the magnet and number of turns in the conductor increases.

ANSWERS TO QUESTIONS

1. Name 3 ways in which a magnetic field can induce a current in a conductor.

   A magnetic field induces an electric current in a conductor when: (1) a conductor is moved across a magnetic field, (2) a magnetic field is moved across a conductor and (3) the strength of the magnetic field in which a conductor lies is increased or decreased without movement of either the magnetizing unit or the conductor relative to the other.

2. What affect does speed of the conductor have on the strength of the current?

   Increasing the speed increases the current.

3. What effect does the number of turns of the conductor have on current?

   The more the turns, the greater the current.

7

OHM'S LAW

Prior to performing this laboratory, the student should have tested competent in the Resistors, Multitesters and Electrical symbols and diagrams laboratories.

As a double check of and reinforcement to the researcher's results, the quantity which is calculated (potential in experiment number 1 and current in experiment number 2) can also be measured. Then the measured value (in volts or amperes) can be compared with the calculated value. The measured and calculated values should be within 5% – 10% of each other. If this is not true, check to make sure the experimenter read the meter correctly, determined the ohms properly and that the mA reading was correctly translated into amperes.

EQUIPMENT

It is recommended that the resistor be a minimum of 120 ohms to avoid overheating of the circuit. If overheating occurs, touching the resistor for any length of time may cause a minor burn. To cool a hot resistor, open the circuit, i.e., take one of the batteries out of the holder.

The equipment used in this laboratory may be obtained inexpensively at electrical or hardware stores. For information on how to build a circuit board, refer to "How to build a circuit board" in the front of this guide.

EXPERIMENTS 1 AND 2

PROCEDURE

If there are not enough circuit boards, the researcher can construct 1 circuit at a time rather than both at once. Also, the order in which the experiments are performed is insignificant as both are autonomous.

Care should be taken to select the correct amount of ohms. Too high a resistance will produce a current so small, it may not be measurable. Too low a resistance may produce such a high current that the resistor burns out. An overloaded circuit is easily detectable by the odor of the burning resistor. If this occurs, do not touch the resistor while it is hot. Open the circuit (remove a battery) and remove the resistor after it cools down.

D A T A

The data depend on the energy of the batteries and amount of resistance selected. Common errors occur when the researcher does not properly change mA to A and misreads or miscalculates the resistor color code.

C O N C L U S I O N FOR EXPERIMENT 1

Ohm's law may be used to determine the amount of voltage of a circuit if the resistance and current are known.

C O N C L U S I O N FOR EXPERIMENT 2

Ohm's law may be used to determine the amount of current of a circuit if the resistance and voltage are known.

ANSWERS TO QUESTIONS

1. Define Ohm's law.

   Ohm's law states that current is directly related to potential and inversely related to resistance.

2. If the voltage is a constant, what happens to the value of the current flow (amperes) when the resistance is increased? What type of relationship would amperes have to resistance in such a case?

   The current decreases. The relationship is inversely proportional.

3. What unit is used to measure potential?

   Potential is measured in volts.

4. What unit is used to measure current?

   Current is measured in amperes.

5. What unit is used to measure resistance?

   Ohms is used to measure resistance.

8

SERIES

CIRCUITS

Prior to performing this laboratory, the student should have tested competent in the Resistors, Multitesters, Ohm's law and Electrical symbols and diagrams laboratories.

EQUIPMENT

It is recommended that the resistors be a minimum of 120 ohms to avoid overheating of the circuit. If overheating occurs, touching the resistor for any length of time may cause a minor burn. To cool a hot resistor, open the circuit, i.e., take one of the batteries out of the holder.

The equipment used in this laboratory may be obtained inexpensively at electrical or hardware stores. For information on how to build a circuit board, refer to "How to build a circuit board" in the front of this guide.

EXPERIMENT 1

PROCEDURE

Unless a fairly sensitive multitester is used, the resistors in this experiment should be within 200 ohms of each other. Using resistors which have a large difference in resistance (e.g., 600 ohms) may result in there being a large variance in potential drop from one resistor to the other. A meter which is capable of measuring only large amounts of milliamperes might not be able to record a current flow in such a situation.

The measured I and R_t, when multiplied together, should be within 3% of the total voltage reading, E_t. If this is not the case, check to make sure that the researcher read the meter correctly and that the milliampere reading was correctly translated into amperes.

D A T A

The readings result in the same mA reading regardless of the meter position. Voltage reading will vary relative to the resistance and in accordance with Ohm's law.

C O N C L U S I O N

Current in a series circuit is constant. The voltage varies relative to the resistance and in accordance with Ohm's law.

E X P E R I M E N T   2

P R O C E D U R E

It is suggested that, instead of connecting both light bulbs to the circuit and disconnecting one bulb, all but one wire be connected to the circuit. The loose wire may be connected to the circuit manually by placing the wire on the appropriate screw connection (make sure to hold the wire by the insulation) or by using a switch. With this method, it is possible to disconnect and reconnect the circuit to observe and re-observe the results several times within a short period of time.

To be able to observe the effect of disconnecting the light bulb, make sure that the intensity of the bulb is sufficient to enable its light to be visualized in a lighted room. If the light is not visualized, it may be possible to visualize the light by dimming the room lights. If the light bulb doesn't illuminate, make sure that the bulb hasn't burned out and that the voltage and amperage required for the bulb are appropriate for the circuit.

V I S U A L   O B S E R V A T I O N

When the light was removed, all lights went out (were not illuminated).

C O N C L U S I O N

If one item in a series circuit does not conduct an electric current, none of the other items in the circuit will receive current, and therefore the circuit will not operate.

ANSWERS TO QUESTIONS

1. What is the relationship of the total current in a two-resistor series circuit to the current passing through r_1 and r_2?

   The total current is the same as the current passing through r_1 and r_2.

2. How is the total resistance of a series circuit calculated?

   The total resistance may be calculated using one of the following formulas:

$$R_t = r_1 + r_2 + \ldots r_n$$

or

$$R_t = E_t/I$$

3. What formula may be used to calculate the total voltage in a series circuit having four resistors?

Total voltage may be calculated using one of the following formulas:

$$E_t = e_1 + e_2 + e_3 + e_4$$

or

$$E_t = IR_t$$

4. What are two advantages of using a series circuit?

Two advantages are in a case of current overload, burnout of a single resistor will stop current flow in the circuit, thereby preventing further damage to the circuit; and voltage across each resistor can be reduced by adding resistors to prevent overloads from occurring in the first place.

9

PARALLEL

CIRCUITS

Prior to performing this laboratory, the student should have tested competent in the Resistors, Multitesters, Ohm's law and Electrical symbols and diagrams laboratories.

EQUIPMENT

The equipment used in this laboratory may be obtained inexpensively at electrical or hardware stores. For information on how to build a circuit board, refer to "How to build a circuit board" in the front of this guide.

The measured I_t and R_t, when multiplied together, should be within 3% of the total voltage reading. If this is not the case, check to make sure that the researcher read the meter correctly and that the milliampere reading was correctly translated into amperes.

EXPERIMENT 1

DATA

The readings result in the same voltage reading regardless of the meter position. Current readings will vary relative to the resistance and in accordance with Ohm's law.

CONCLUSION

Voltage in a series circuit is constant. The current varies relative to the resistance and in accordance with Ohm's law.

E X P E R I M E N T   2

P R O C E D U R E

It is suggested that, instead of connecting both light bulbs to the circuit and disconnecting one bulb, all but one wire be connected to the circuit. The loose wire may be connected to the circuit manually by placing the wire on the appropriate screw connection (make sure to hold wire by the insulation) or by using a switch. With this method, it is possible to disconnect and reconnect the circuit to observe and re-observe the results several times within a short period of time.

To be able to observe the effect of disconnecting the light bulb, make sure that the intensity of the bulb is sufficient to enable its light to be visualized in a lighted room. If the light is not visualized, it may be possible to visualize the light by dimming the room lights. If the light bulb doesn't illuminate, make sure that the bulb hasn't burned out and that the voltage and amperage required for the bulb are appropriate for the circuit.

V I S U A L   O B S E R V A T I O N

When the light was removed, all lights remaining in the circuit were still lit (were illuminated).

C O N C L U S I O N

If one item in a parallel circuit does not conduct an electric current, all the other items in the circuit will receive current, and therefore, the circuit will continue to operate.

ANSWERS TO QUESTIONS

1. What relationship does the total voltage in a 2 resistor parallel circuit have to the voltages across r_1 and r_2?

   The voltage is the same over r_1 and r_2.

2. How is the total resistance calculated in a parallel circuit?

   The total resistance (R_t) is inversely proportional to the sum of the reciprocal of the individual resistances. This is represented mathematically as

   $$1/R_t = 1/r_1 + 1/r_2 + \ldots . 1/r_n$$

   By algebraic rules, it is possible to employ Ohm's law to determine the formula for R_t. The result is

   $$R_t = r_1 r_2 \ldots r n/(r_1 + r_2 + \ldots r_n)$$

   or

   $$R_t = E/I_t$$

3. Express in words and in a formula an equivalent for the total current (I_t) in a parallel circuit having 4 resistors.

   The total current is the sum of the individual currents over the 4 resistors.

   The formula is: $I_t = i_1 + i_2 + i_3 + i_4$

10

STEP UP AND STEP DOWN TRANS- FORMERS

Prior to performing this laboratory, the student should have tested competent in the Multitesters and Electrical symbols and diagrams laboratories.

EQUIPMENT

The equipment used in this laboratory may be obtained inexpensively at electrical or hardware stores. For information on how to build a circuit board, refer to "How to build a circuit board" in the front of this guide.

EXPERIMENT 1

PROCEDURE

For safety purposes, the potential of the wall socket need not be measured. The potential may be recorded as 110 volts. However, it is entirely possible that the potential is slightly higher or lower than 110 volts. If this is true, the transformer ratio may not appear to be the same as the ratio labelled on the transformer by the manufacturer. Also, if some of the energy produced by the transformer is in the form of heat, the manufacturers's transformer ratio will appear to be "off."

DATA

The voltage on the secondary side should be lower than the primary side. The amount of decrease is directly proportional to the ratio of the transformer.

CONCLUSION

The transformer constructed was a step down transformer. The effective voltage on the secondary side was lower than the primary side. The amount of decrease was directly related to the transformer ratio.

EXPERIMENT 2

PROCEDURE

Transformers produce heat, which results in an electrical energy or power loss (law of conservation of energy). This loss will cause a lower than projected voltage output, the result being that the measured effective transformer ratio may not be the same as the ratio labelled on the transformer by the manufacturer.

The voltage on the secondary side may be fairly high (110). Thus, **do not** allow the experimenters to touch the secondary wires when the circuit is closed.

DATA

The voltage on the secondary side should be higher than the primary side. The amount of increase is directly proportional to the ratio of the transformer.

CONCLUSION

The transformer constructed was a step up transformer. The voltage on the secondary side was higher than the primary side and the increase was directly related to the transformer ratio.

ANSWERS TO QUESTIONS

1. What is the theoretical transformer ratio?

   The theoretical transformer ratio is the ratio of the number of turns in the secondary coil, N_s, to the number of turns in the primary coil, N_p.

2. What is the effective transformer ratio?

   The effective transformer ratio is the ratio of the electromotive force (voltage) of the secondary coil, E_s, to the electromotive force of the primary coil, E_p.

3. What effect did the step-down transformer have on voltage?

   Voltage was decrease relative to the ratio of the transformer.

4. What effect did the step-up transformer have on voltage?

   Voltage was increased relative to the ratio of the transformer.

11

TRANSFORMER POWER AND EFFICIENCY

Prior to performing this laboratory, the student should have tested competent in the Resistors, Multitesters and Electrical symbols and diagrams laboratories.

EQUIPMENT

The equipment used in this laboratory may be obtained inexpensively at electrical or hardware stores. For information on how to build a circuit board, refer to "How to build a circuit board" in the front of this guide.

DATA

The experimenter should accurately record all data and calculate the power and efficiency.

CONCLUSION

The experimenter should be able to summarize the power of the primary and secondary sides of the transformer as well as its efficiency. However, it should be noted that although most texts identify transformer efficiency as 90%, the experience of the authors is that when dealing with transformers of the size in this laboratory, the efficiency may be as low as 35%.

Since energy cannot be created or destroyed, the researcher should not have an efficiency over 100%.

ANSWERS TO QUESTIONS

1. State the law of conservation of energy.

   The conservation of energy law states that energy may be converted from one form to another but energy may be neither created nor destroyed.

2. Give at least 3 formulas that may be used to express power in a transformer circuit.

   Three formulas for power are: $P = IE$, $P = E^2/R$ and $P = I^2R$

3. What is the formula for transformer efficiency?

   The formula for efficiency is: Efficiency = P_s/P_p x 100

4. List at least 2 reasons why the efficiency was less than 100%.

   Factors that result in the efficiency being less than 100% include: electrical currents induced in the core, magnetic field reactions and differences in resistance between the primary and secondary coils.

12

RECTIFICATION

Prior to performing this laboratory, the student should have tested competent in the Multitesters, Resistors and Electrical Symbols and Diagrams laboratories.

EQUIPMENT

The equipment and materials used in this laboratory may be obtained from electrical and hardware stores. For information on how to build your own circuit board, refer to the "How to Build a Circuit Board" section of this instructor's guide.

PROCEDURE

The small work area of the circuit board described in this manual may make the construction of full wave rectified circuits cumbersome and difficult. To eliminate this problem it is recommended that the wires from the 4 required diodes be soldered together and then connected to the terminal strip. Figure 12–1 represents the correct way to connect the diodes. It is important to note the direction of the diodes (note the location of the "band" around the diode) and the location of the wires. The wires labeled "A" are attached to the resistor on the terminal and the wires labeled "B" are connected to the secondary side of the step down transformer.

It is recommended that the researcher construct the circuit leaving the step to connect the transformer to the wall socket last. Prior to the experimenter plugging in the transformer, the instructor should inspect the circuit.

The experimenter may discover that both an AC and DC voltage can be measured at the leads coming from the rectifier(s). This results from 1 or more of the following conditions:

a. There is some AC leakage past the rectifier diodes.

b. The AC voltmeter consists of a moving coil, a diode and a permanent magnet which react to the pulsating direct current from the rectifier.

c. The AC voltmeter consists of a moving coil and a field coil. The magnetic fields of the coils react with each other by the transformer principle regardless of the current direction.

Because this laboratory concentrates on DC voltage, the AC voltage measurements have been ignored to avoid confusion. It is left to the discretion of the instructor whether to include the concept of AC voltage.

If the measurements do not support the rectifier theory, check to see that the multitester is set up properly and that the readings have been recorded accurately.

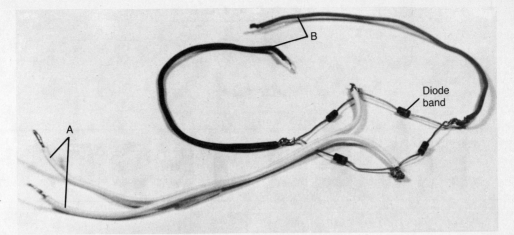

Figure 12–1. Correct way to solder 4 diodes and connecting wires for full wave rectification.

DATA

Since the incoming voltage is alternating, the researcher should not measure DC or direct current in the unrectified circuit. The DC voltage measurement in the half wave rectified circuit should be approximately half the DC voltage measured in the full wave rectified circuit.

CONCLUSION

The measured potential difference (volts) demonstrates that it is possible to change the direction of alternating current to direct current. The type of rectification determines the amount of potential available.

ANSWERS TO QUESTIONS

1. Define rectification.

   Rectification is the conversion of alternating current to direct current.

2. What electrical components may be used to achieve rectification?

   Rectification can be accomplished by inverters (electromechanical devices), electronic diode tubes, electrolytic devices and semiconductor diodes (solid-state rectifiers).

3. How many positive pulses occur in 1 second in a half wave rectified single phase alternating current with a frequency of 60 cps?

   There are 60 positive or useful pulses per second in a half wave rectified 60 cps single phase alternating current.

13

TIMER TESTS

There are 3 noninvasive methods described in this laboratory that may be employed to test an x-ray timer. It is suggested that the experimenter perform only 1 of the 3 methods. However, the procedures are brief enough to allow the student to perform all of them within a normal 3 hour laboratory session. If the researcher performs 1 of the 3 procedures, the instructor may wish to divide the class into at least 3 groups having each group perform a different method. The groups may then meet to exchange information to introduce them to the various methods.

SPINNING TOP

PROCEDURE

This procedure is best performed with a minimum of 2 experimenters. One person spins the top while the other makes the exposure. The instructor is encouraged to remind the students that no exposure is to be made until the person spinning the top is clear of the radiation field.

The speed of the top regulates the length of the dots and the distance between them. If the top rotates too fast or too slow, the dots superimpose one another making it impossible to assess the radiograph. Also, too many dots result in overlap. Thus, it is recommended that a time no longer than 1/10 second be used for self or half wave rectified x-ray units and 1/20 second for full wave rectified units. Since self and half wave units are uncommon, this laboratory is written for full wave rectified machines. To obtain a sufficient amount of dots on the radiograph, schools with half or self wave rectified machines may wish to use 1/10 and 1/15 second exposure.

A spinning top may also be used to assess rectifier failure. This is identified on a radiograph as alternating light and dark dots. This laboratory is designed to limit the use of the spinning top to timer assessment. However, the instructor may wish to introduce rectifier malfunction information.

VISUAL OBSERVATIONS

The type of information located in this section is a summary of the findings relative to the density of the dots. Instructors including assessment of the rectifiers should advise students to include their findings regarding dot densities in this section.

It is not unusual for experimenters to also include the number of dots in this section. The instructor may wish to consider advising the student that the number of dots is more appropriately placed in the data section.

SYNCHRONOUS MOTOR

P R O C E D U R E

A synchronous motor is designed to assess both milliampere and time. The milliampere is evaluated by using a penetrometer located at the bottom of the test tool, below the disc. Since a milliampere assessment is located in the Milliampere Check laboratory, it is recommended that the instructor have the experimenter cone to the disc only. This limits the information on the radiograph to timer assessment.

Synchronous motors need electricity to operate. Therefore, the instructor should check the location of the electrical outlet relative to the x-ray tube and table prior to performing this laboratory. It may be possible that an extension cord is needed to allow the motor to be plugged in the wall socket.

C O N C L U S I O N

Specific conclusion comments depend on the method employed to assess the timer. The spinning top procedure conclusion should address the number of dots obtained on the radiograph relative to the number of dots calculated. In other words, are the dots within plus or minus 1 indicating the timer is acceptable. The density should also be addressed. The student should be able to determine if the time is starting and stopping at the correct portion of the sine wave. Students required to assess rectifier function should indicate their status in this section.

The synchronous motor test conclusion for single phase units is the same as the spinning top test. The difference being, it is impractical to assess slit density. On three phase equipment, the experimenter should relate the angle of the image to timer accuracy.

The digital testing tool is probably the simplest method, especially if the instrument is set to readout specific time vs. impulses. The researcher should correlate the readout with the time set to determine the accuracy of the time.

ANSWERS TO QUESTIONS

1. How many dots should be produced on a spinning top radiograph by a single phase, half wave rectified, 60 cps x-ray unit utilizing 300 mA, 60 kV and 1/30 second exposure (show math)?

   $$\text{number of dots} = \text{exposure time} \times \text{cps} \times \text{useful impulses/cycle}$$

   $$X = 1/30 \times 60 \times 1$$

   $$x = 2 \text{ dots}$$

2. List 2 things influencing the number of impulses used by timers.

   the type of rectification

   the type of timer used

   the type of current entering the machine

3. List two types of noninvasive tools used to check the accuracy of a timer.

   Noninvasive timer test tools are spinning top, synchronous timer and digital test tool.

4. A test is done on a three phase x-ray unit. The time used is 1/10 second. The arc on the radiograph measures 42 degrees. Is the timer working properly? Why or why not.

   The acceptable angle range for the given technique is 33-40.7 or

$$\text{degrees} = (\text{time used} \times 360) + 1 \text{ degree}$$

$$X = 1/10 \times 360 + 1$$

$$= 36 + 1$$

$$= 37$$

Acceptable limit is plus or minus 10%

$$37 \times 0.10 = 3.7$$

$$\text{lower limit} = 37 - 3.7 = 33$$

$$\text{upper limit} = 37 + 3.7 = 40.7$$

A measured angle of 42 is outside the acceptable range.

5. While using a digital timer testing tool, an exposure is made and the red LED illuminates. What can be done to adjust technique so the red LED will not illuminate?

A red LED indicates x-ray intensity over range, thus a need exists to decrease the milliampere or kilovoltage.

14

DENSITY AND EXPOSURE MEASURING DEVICES

This laboratory is designed to acquaint the researcher with the various types of density and exposure instruments associated with the laboratory experiments of this manual. The most common instruments used are densitometer and penetrometer. At least 3 laboratories, Milliampere check, Half value layer and Inverse square law, employ a dosimeter pencil and charger or other similar exposure measuring devices.

The type of equipment owned by schools is often determined by the amount of their budget relative to equipment costs and maintenance. Most radiography schools tend to own a densitometer and penetrometer. However, fewer schools tend to possess a dosimeter pencil and charger. The instructor should modify this laboratory to match the type of equipment the student will be using.

EXPERIMENT 1: DENSITOMETER

PROCEDURE

There are several types of densitometers on the market. Most read in logarithm (log) while others read both log (density) and percent (transmissivity). It is not unusual for schools to own more than one type of densitometer. The student should become familiar with all types of densitometers that may be used during the semester or term.

The design of the densitometer determines the maximum film size that can be read. Some densitometers can only read about 7 inches of a radiograph. These densitometers are small and handy to use. They are most useful in reading sensitometry films. However, they are impractical for measuring densities of large radiographs.

The instructor may either supply a radiograph with several density shades or have the student take a radiograph of an object to obtain several densities. Regardless of whether the instructor or student obtains the radiograph, care needs to be taken to insure the densitometer can accommodate the film size.

CONCLUSION

The student should be able to identify the location of the light source and photoelectric cell of the densitometer. If more than one type of densitometer is used, the researcher should briefly explain the differences. Lastly, the experimenter is expected to be able to identify the purpose of a densitometer: to read radiographic density.

EXPERIMENT 2: DOSIMETER PENCIL

PROCEDURE

Since dosimeter pencils have a fairly high error range, it is important that an average of 3 exposure readings be taken. Also, care should be taken to employ dosimeter pencils which can measure the radiation output of the x-ray machine. Dosimeters that read in RADS may not be sensitive enough to deflect the hairline due to low energy output of the x-ray machine.

CONCLUSION

The conclusion should contain a comment that a dosimeter pencil is used to measure radiation exposure. The experimenter may note that there was a minor difference among any 3 exposures using the same technique. The differences may be attributed to the level of accuracy of the dosimeter or equipment fluctuation.

EXPERIMENT 3: PENETROMETER

VISUAL OBSERVATION

This section contains information the experimenter observes. Namely, that the density of the steps decreased in darkness as the numbers on the penetrometer increased.

CONCLUSION

The conclusion is derived from the observation, in other words, the "cause" of the difference in densities. Thus, the student should conclude that the thick part of the penetrometer absorbed more radiation creating a lighter image. The experimenter may also be able to reason that from the difference in density, a penetrometer can measure the penetrability of an x-ray beam in matter.

Sometimes the student puts the conclusion in the observation section. This tends to create confusion as is often demonstrated by the student's inability to write an appropriate conclusion. Thus, it is recommended that the instructor advise the student of the different type of information expected for the observation and conclusion.

ANSWERS TO QUESTIONS

1. What does a densitometer measure?

   A densitometer is an instrument for measuring optical density of a radiograph.

2. What are the major components of a typical densitometer?

   The typical densitometer consists of a light source, photoelectric cell and electronics used to indicate the density on a scale.

3. What does a dosimeter pencil measure?

   A dosimeter is a device from which radiation exposure may be measured and radiation dose inferred.

4. What does a penetrometer measure?

   A penetrometer is a device used for determining the relative penetrability of an x-ray beam in matter.

5. What is a common name for a penetrometer?

   Penetrometer is commonly referred to as a step-wedge.

15

AUTOMATIC TIMERS

EXPERIMENT 1

VISUAL OBSERVATION

The density should appear about the same for both radiographs.

CONCLUSION

Assuming the density appeared the same, the automatic timer is functioning properly. Also, the experimenter may conclude that the automatic timer produces the same density for an object of the same composition but different thickness. If the densities in the visual observation section were not similar, then the student must present possible reasons for the differences.

EXPERIMENT 2

DATA

Although it is not possible to provide the specific numerical exposure values the researcher will experience, this section should demonstrate that the exposure time decreased as the kVp increased.

VISUAL OBSERVATION

The contrast should have decreased (more shades of gray, long scale) as the kVp increased.

CONCLUSION

As the kVp increased, the exposure time and contrast decreased due to an increase in remnant radiation. If the data section did not demonstrate an exposure time decrease or the densities in the visual observation section were not similar, then the student must present possible reasons for the differences.

ANSWERS TO QUESTIONS

1. Define automatic timer.

   Automatic exposure timers provide automatic control of radiographic exposure by terminating the exposure when the quantity of the remnant beam reaches a preselected value.

2. What effect does kVp have on the exposure time?

   As the kVp increases, the exposure time decreases.

3. How is the density of a radiograph increased when using an automatic timer?

   The radiographic density is changed by adjusting the density knob located on the x-ray machine control panel. This adjusts the amount of remnant radiation needed to automatically terminate the exposure.

4. What is the purpose of the radiation detectors on an automatic timer?

   A radiation detector is employed to measure the radiation and "send" a message to terminate the exposure.

16

FOCAL

SPOT SIZE

This laboratory may be performed in several different ways (with a pinhole camera, a test star pattern or homemade equipment). Instructors must determine which method or methods are most appropriate for their school. Experimenters may learn more if each group uses different methods of performing this experiment and the results of the different methods are compared at the end of the laboratory session.

PROCEDURE

It is important to know the exact location of the x-ray tube target. The target location is needed to determine the enlargement factor of the radiographic image. If the target location is known and the 1:1 ratio is used, no enlargement factor adjustment is needed. However, if the location of the focal spot is unknown, it is nearly impossible to obtain a 1:1 ratio. In this case, the enlargement factor must be calculated.

To calculate the ratio, drill one hole in the metal plate 0.70 cm to the left of the pinhole. Drill a second hole 0.70 cm to the right of the pinhole. This results in a 1.4 cm distance between the holes.

Radiograph the plate as indicated in the experiment. Measure the distance between the 2 side holes on the radiograph. Determine the enlargement factor by using the following formula:

image measurement$/1.40$ = enlargement factor

For example, if the distance between the 2 side holes in the radiographic image is 1.86 cm, the enlargement factor is approximately $1.86/1.40 = 1.33$.

This means that a focal spot which measured 2.66 mm on the radiograph would have an actual size of $2.66/1.33 = 2.00$ mm.

DATA

The data depend on the type of x-ray tube and the size and shape of the filament.

VISUAL OBSERVATION

A normal focal spot demonstrates a rectangle shape which has a fairly sharp image. The larger focal spot demonstrates more penumbra or unsharpness. If any irregularities occur in the size or shape of the image, it may indicate a problem with the target or filament.

CONCLUSION

The conclusion is directly related to the data and visual observation findings. In general, this section should contain information about the size and shape of the focal spots. The experimenter should provide possible reasons for any image irregularities.

ANSWERS TO QUESTIONS

1. Define effective and true focal spot.

   The true focal spot size is the area of the anode target upon which the electron beam impinges. The effective focal spot represents the apparent size of the true focal spot when it is viewed from underneath on a line of sight perpendicular to the flow of electrons.

2. What effect does a change in the size of the focal spot have on geometric image quality?

   Increasing the focal spot size decreases geometric image quality.

3. Although reducing the true focal spot size improves radiographic image quality, why might it sometimes be impractical to use the smallest focal spot size on the x-ray unit?

   If the focal spot size is too small to handle a given technique, it tends to produce a large amount of heat at the anode and electrolysis which can be destructive to the target.

HEEL EFFECT

EQUIPMENT

To avoid any variation in radiographic density created by factors other than the heel effect, e.g., intensifying screens, a direct film holder is used. This laboratory identifies the need for 3 direct film holders. If there are not enough film holders for the class, then 1 holder may be employed. However, if 1 film holder is used, it must be reloaded after every exposure. The size of the film holder is important. Since the heel effect depends upon field size, it is best to employ a large film (14″ x 17″) for optimum results.

PROCEDURE

The amount of density on the radiograph is important. Too much or too little density will not demonstrate the heel effect. Therefore, it is strongly recommended that a density between 0.7 and 1.0 be employed.

When measuring density, it is important to avoid measuring penumbra. Also, to prevent the lead letters or numbers from interfering with the density readings, they should be positioned several inches from the film edge.

The instructor should advise the student to be careful when taking measurements. The longitudinal density is obtained by measuring midline of the 17 inch portion of the radiograph. The cathode and anode readings are measured along the respective 14 inch side of the radiograph.

The following is an example of how to calculate percent. Given a 7 inch longitudinal reading of 1.0 and an 8 inch reading of 1.04, the percent for 8 inches is 104% or

$$1.04 / 1.00 \times 100 = 104\%$$

CONCLUSION

There are three points to mention in this laboratory. One is that the cathode end of all radiographs demonstrated a higher reading than the anode edge. This illustrates the concept of the heel effect in which the beam intensity is greater toward the cathode end of the film. Another element in the conclusion is that the heel effect is more noticeable at a short SID. The last item is that large field sizes demonstrate a more pronounced heel effect.

ANSWERS TO QUESTIONS

1. What is the heel effect?

   The heel effect is an uneven distribution of radiation intensity caused when some of the x-ray generated by electrons impinging on the anode are absorbed by the anode itself.

2. How is the beam intensity distributed in the heel effect?

   The heel effect results in more radiation being emitted toward the cathode.

3. What effect does source image distance have on the heel effect?

   The heel effect is more prevalent when employing a short source image distance.

4. What effect does field size have on the heel effect?

   The heel effect is more prevalent when employing a large field size.

5. When is the heel effect disadvantageous?

   The heel effect is a disadvantage when radiographing an object having a relatively uniform density, e.g., wrist.

6. When might the heel effect be used to an advantage?

   The heel effect is advantageous when a structure is more opaque on one side than the other, e.g., anterior-posterior thoracic spine.

18

KILOVOLTAGE COMPEN-SATION

EQUIPMENT

Since this experiment is very dependent on the photographic aspect of the image, it is important to limit external factors which may influence density or contrast. Consequently, a direct film holder is employed.

Also, the laboratory requires the manipulation of kilovoltage, milliampere and time. Thus, equipment permitting manual setting of techniques is needed. Units with automatic timing mechanisms do not permit the manual adjustment of the milliampere and time.

PROCEDURE

Since the kilovoltage is varied in this experiment, it is important to employ a phantom part which requires no less than 75 kilovolts to obtain a diagnostic radiograph for the original film. If lower kV values are used, the latitude is greatly reduced.

It is important to encourage the experimenter to maintain the same focal spot size (FSS) when altering the mAs. It is possible that a change in FSS may affect the photographic quality of the image.

VISUAL OBSERVATION

All 3 radiographs should display a diagnostic "readable" radiograph. However, the change in kilovoltage demonstrates an obvious change in contrast. Lower kilovoltages display a higher contrast. It is possible to amend the laboratory to include a penetrometer on the film. The penetrometer is useful in illustrating the effect on contrast.

CONCLUSION

The experimenter should be able to conclude that it is possible to alter the technique by using the 13% and 15% kilovoltage compensation rules. The result is a comparable diagnostic radiograph with evidence of contrast changes.

ANSWERS TO QUESTIONS

1. List 2 methods which may be employed for setting technical factors.

   Two methods employed for setting technical factors are the manual method and the automatic exposure timer technique.

2. What does the operator adjust when employing an automatic timer x-ray unit?

   The operator adjusts the kilovoltage.

3. A radiograph is taken at 75 kV, 300 mA and 0.10 seconds. The radiograph must be repeated using 1/2 the mAs. What new technical factors may be employed to obtain approximately the same quality as the original radiograph? (Show all math)

   Original mAs = 300 x 0.10 = 30

   New technique = 15 mAs (any mA and s combination to = 15 mAs) and 86 kilovolts (75 x 0.15 = 11.25, 75 + 11 = 86)

KILOVOLTAGE CHECK

This laboratory requires the use of a commercial kVp assessment cassette. Most cassettes are constructed to test both kVp and Half Value Layer, HVL. This laboratory concentrates on the assessment of kilovoltage. One common cassette is distributed by the Radiation Measurement Instruments (RMI), Wisconsin cassette. The instructor should be advised that the Wisconsin cassette is more accurate at low kilovoltage than high kilovoltage. This is especially true with cassettes manufactured prior to 1982. Also, since the cassette measures peak kilovoltage and electrical variations influence the kilovoltage value, the Wisconsin cassette is more accurate when a 3 phase x-ray unit is employed. Although either blue sensitive or green sensitive film may be employed with the cassette, there are minor variations in results. Thus, it is recommended that the cassette be calibrated to coincide with the film most often used in the department. To maximize the results, it is also recommended that the cassette be calibrated every 2 years. Cassettes may be calibrated by sending them to the National Bureau of Standards in Washington, D. C. or the University of Wisconsin Radiation Calibration Service (UWRCS) in Madison, Wisconsin.

DATA

The information located in this section depends upon the accuracy of the x-ray machine.

CONCLUSION

The conclusion depends upon the results found in the data. In general, the experimenter should be able to determine if the x-ray machine's kVp output is within the acceptable range.

ANSWERS TO QUESTIONS

1. On what principle or concept is a wide range cassette based?

   The design for the cassette is based upon Ardan and Crooke's cassette. Their cassette is designed to take advantage of the concept that the rate of attenuation of a heavily filtered x-ray beam is similar to the kilovoltage applied to the x-ray tube. Thus, the cassette is designed to attenuate the x-ray beam.

2. What radiographic effect may occur if the applied kilovoltage is 7 kVp greater than the set kVp?

The result is increased penetration of the object and decreased contrast (more shades of gray).

3. What is the acceptable kilovoltage range for 80 kVp? Show math.

The acceptable range is approximately 78 - 82 kVp.

$$0.03 \times 80 = 2.4$$

$$80 - 2.4 = 77.6$$

$$80 + 2.4 = 82.4$$

4. If a test was performed using 60 kVp on a 3 phase x-ray machine and the matching step was 3, is the equipment operating within the acceptable limits? Why or why not? (Refer to appropriate graph supplied by the cassette manufacturer.)

If the graph exceeds the acceptable range for 60 kVp, the machine is not operating properly.

HALF VALUE
LAYER

PROCEDURE

This laboratory may be performed in several different ways, with commercial equipment (e.g., RMI Test kit), graphically or mathematically. If commercial equipment is used, follow the instructions provided with the equipment.

If an R-meter is used, the scale of the meter must be positioned so that it is easily read from the control area during the exposure. Scintillation counters are sensitive instruments. If the counter readings are erratic, the detector may be too sensitive and need to be shielded by covering the probe with lead.

Different x-ray machines have different outputs. If readings cannot be obtained with the recommended techniques, adjust the technique to accommodate the equipment being used.

Make sure to remove any added filtration before beginning the experiment. Check the information that came with the x-ray tube to determine the inherent filtration rate.

CONCLUSION

The researcher should be able to identify the HVL for each kVp employed. Also, the experimenter should conclude that as the kVp increased there was an increase in HVL and beam quality.

ANSWERS TO QUESTIONS

1. Define "half-value layer."

   HVL is the amount of thickness of a particular material required to reduce the beam intensity by one-half.

2. What material is most commonly used to determine the HVL for diagnostic x-ray?

   The most common material is aluminum.

3. What happens to HVL as kilovoltage increases?

   As kVp increases, the HVL increases.

21

EFFECT OF
KILOVOLTAGE
ON CONTRAST

EQUIPMENT

This laboratory calls for the use of cardboard film holders. If cardboard film holders and nonscreen film are not available, it is recommended that high resolution intensifying screen film holders and film be used. Replacing the cardboard film holder with a cassette (intensifying screen) and/or screen film introduces a loss of radiographic quality resulting from the film emulsion and the construction and composition of the intensifying screen. Thus, the effect of kilovoltage on contrast may be distorted.

Some x-ray machines may not allow for increases in kilovolts by increments of four. The number of kilovolts increased from one exposure to the next exposure is not significant. However, it is important to continually increase the kilovoltage from one exposure to the next (a minimum of a 10% kVp increase is recommended).

VISUAL OBSERVATION

The contrast (difference between the image and the surrounding area of the image) decreases from the first to last exposure.

CONCLUSION

Contrast decreases as the kilovoltage increases.

ANSWERS TO QUESTIONS

1. Define radiographic contrast.

Radiographic contrast is defined as the difference between the radiographic density (darkness) of the field which surrounds the image of the object and the radiographic density (darkness) of the object's image; the greater the difference between the density of the field and the density of the object's image, the higher the contrast.

2. What effect does increasing kilovoltage have on an x-ray beam's ability to penetrate an object?

   As kVp increases there is an increase in the ability of the x-ray beam to penetrate the object.

3. What effect does increasing kilovoltage have on contrast?

   Increasing kVp decreases contrast.

22

MILLIAMPERE

CHECK

There are 3 tests or experiments associated with this laboratory: mA consistency, linear relationship of mA and reproducibility. All the experiments may be performed by using either a dosimeter pencil or penetrometer. Each experiment has two procedures. One procedure represents the steps needed to perform the test if employing a dosimeter pencil, the other procedure is written for using a penetrometer as the testing tool. Follow the instruction manual when using the multi-function meter.

The 3 experiments assess different aspects of mA or mAs. Thus, it is recommended that the student perform all the experiments. However, the researcher needs to perform only 1 of the procedures listed under the experiment. If a choice exists as to which procedure to perform, it is recommended to use either the dosimeter pencil or multi-function meter method. These methods remove some of the variables which may affect the experiment, e.g., processor.

DETERMINING PERCENT DIFFERENCE

The calculations for determining the percent difference for the penetrometer and dosimeter results are similar. Therefore, only one example is provided here.

The first step is to determine which reading is to be used as the standard. This laboratory arbitrarily selected exposure 2 as the standard. Instructors may wish to select a standard other than exposure 2. After selecting the standard, 1 of the remaining 2 exposure readings is subtracted from the standard. To avoid negative numbers, the lower value is subtracted from the higher value. Then the result is divided by the standard. The following is a mathematical example.

	Density Reading	Percent Difference
Exposure 1	1.03	3%
Exposure 2 (standard)	1.00	0%
Exposure 3	1.10	10%

Calculation of percent difference between Standard and Exposure 1

$$1.03 - 1.00 = 0.03$$
$$0.03/1.00 \times 100 = 3\%$$

Calculation of percent difference between Standard and Exposure 3

$$1.10 - 1.00 = 0.10$$
$$0.10 / 1.00 \times 100 = 10\%$$

EXPERIMENT 1: CONSISTENCY

CONCLUSION

If a penetrometer was employed for the experiment, then an accurate test demonstrates the respective densities are within 15% of each other. The dosimeter and multi-function meter results should yield readings which are within 10% of each other, respectively.

EXPERIMENT 2: LINEAR RELATIONSHIP OF MILLIAMPERE

CONCLUSION

The penetrometer test results in densities which increase proportional to the mA increase (within 15%). In other words, every time the mA is doubled, there should be an increase in density of 100%. Results for the dosimeter and multi-function meter demonstrate readings which are proportional to the mA increase (within 10%).

EXPERIMENT 3: REPRODUCIBILITY

CONCLUSION

The conclusion for experiment number 3 is the same as experiment number 1.

ANSWERS TO QUESTIONS

1. What is milliampere?

   Milliampere (mA) represents the x-ray tube current.

2. List 2 things that may influence mA test results.

   The variables which influence the mA test results are

   proper function of the automatic processor

   no law of reciprocity failure

   accurate kilovoltage settings

   proper function of the timer

3. What does the mA consistency test check?

The consistency test is used to assess whether or not the mAs output is constant for a given mAs regardless of the mA or time employed.

4. What does the mA linear test assess?

The linear assessment demonstrates density or dose differences which coincide with the milliampere change.

5. What does the mA reproducibility test check?

The reproducibility test is used to determine if a given mAs output is constant from one exposure to the next.

6. What is the advantage of using a dosimeter or multi-function meter vs. penetrometer as the instrument to assess mA?

The dosimeter pencil and multi-function meter are the more accurate milliampere evaluation procedures because they limit the number of variables, e.g., no need to use the processor or film.

23

LAW OF

RECIPROCITY

EQUIPMENT

It is important to use nonscreen holders in this laboratory. Although extremity cassettes have high resolution, the screen produces light when irradiated. This may cause density problems.

PROCEDURE

To limit the heel effect, a long source image distance (SID) is employed. Also, make sure the 3 sections of the film to be exposed are parallel to the longitudinal axis of the x-ray tube. The film should be placed on the x-ray table so the longitudinal axis is perpendicular to the longitudinal axis of the x-ray tube ("transverse" position if the film were placed on the x-ray table). This distributes the heel effect equally over all 3 sections. Placing the longitudinal axis of the film parallel to the longitudinal axis of the x-ray tube results in only one end (section) of the film being exposed to the heel effect.

Another factor influencing density is the focal spot size (FSS). To avoid density changes due to the FSS the milliampere selected to obtain 100 mAs should energize the same focal spot. If it isn't possible to obtain the same FSS for 3 exposures at 100 mAs, select an appropriate mAs to permit the use of the same FSS for 3 exposures.

VISUAL OBSERVATION

The specific information located in this section depends upon the results of the experiment. The student should mention the visual effects among the 3 exposures, e.g., exposures appeared to be of equal density to the human eye. No mention should be made relative to contrast. This is because contrast is the difference between 2 densities and each exposure has only 1 density.

DATA

The first step in calculating the percent density difference is to determine which reading is to be used as the standard. It is recommended that the middle range density be used as the standard. After selecting the standard, 1 of the remaining 2 exposure readings is subtracted from the standard. For example, select the density to be compared to the standard. Subtract the lower density reading from the higher density (this avoids negative numbers). The result is then divided by the standard and multiplied by 100. The following is a mathematical example.

	Density Reading	Percent Difference
Exposure 1	1.03	3%
Exposure 2 (standard)	1.00	0%
Exposure 3	1.10	10%

Calculation of percent difference between Standard and Exposure 1

$$1.03 - 1.00 = 0.03$$
$$0.03/1.00 \times 100 = 3\%$$

Calculation of percent difference between Standard and Exposure 3

$$1.10 - 1.00 = 0.10$$
$$0.10/1.00 \times 100 = 10\%$$

CONCLUSION

The conclusion is dependent upon the radiographic findings. In general, the student should be able to determine if there is a reciprocity law failure by visual observation and the data section. Any change in density by 15% is considered a reciprocity failure.

ANSWERS TO QUESTIONS

1. What does the law of reciprocity state?

   The law of reciprocity for film exposure states that the effective action of radiant exposure is constant when the product of the intensity of the radiance by the elapsed time of the exposure is constant. For radiography, this may be expressed in the form of the following formula.

   $$mAs = mA \times s$$

2. Give 3 examples of the law of reciprocity for 200 mAs.

   There are an infinite number of combinations of mA and s which may be used to obtain 200 mAs. It is suggested that the instructor advise the student to limit the choices to those most commonly found on an x-ray machine.

3. Under what conditions and exposure values is the law of reciprocity apt to fail?

   There is a reciprocity failure when mAs is used with intensifying screens. This reciprocity failure exists at mA and time settings which are at the extreme ends of the exposure range.

4. What is the factor which causes the law of reciprocity to fail?

   Reciprocity law failure is due to the film in the intensifying screen being exposed by light vs. radiation.

24

EFFECT OF MILLIAMPERE-SECONDS ON DENSITY

EQUIPMENT

It is important to use nonscreen holders in this laboratory. Although extremity cassettes have high resolution, the screen produces light when irradiated. This may cause density problems.

VISUAL OBSERVATION

The student should be able to identify that there is an increase in density as the milliampere-seconds increased.

CONCLUSION

The conclusion is very similar to the visual observation in that there is an increase in density as the mAs increases. There is not enough information obtained from this experiment to conclude that there is a direct relationship between density and mAs, e.g., double mAs, double the density. These data may be obtained by taking densitometer measurements of the same step for each exposure and calculating the percent increase.

57

ANSWERS TO QUESTIONS

1. What is mAs?

   Milliampere-seconds is the quantity of electrons that pass from the cathode to the anode (target) of an x-ray tube during the course of an x-ray exposure.

2. What effect does increasing mAs have on the quantity of x-ray produced?

   Increasing mAs for a particular kilovoltage setting (x-ray tube potential) increases the number of x-ray photons (quantity) emitted from the x-ray tube target.

3. What effect does increasing mAs have on radiographic density?

   The greater the mAs, the greater the density (darkness) of the radiographic image of the object.

4. Define radiographic density.

   Density is log opacity (O) or the log incident light/transmitted light. This is represented mathematically as

   $$D = \log O = \log I_o / I_t$$

25

TOMOGRAPHY: FULCRUM LEVEL

EQUIPMENT

Since this laboratory requires the experimenter to take 5 tomographic sections, an angle block of sufficient height to accommodate 5 levels must be employed. Also, it is best if the block contain numbers (in centimeter increments) which coincide with the fulcrum level set, e.g., if a level of 5 cm is set, the block should demonstrate the number 5 on the tomogram.

PROCEDURE

A small exposure angle should be employed. This creates a thin tomographic section facilitating the ability of the experimenter to determine the relationship between the set fulcrum level and image quality. A thick tomographic section may visualize more than 1 centimeter of clarity.

When setting the fulcrum level, due to the parallax effect, the experimenter's eye level must be perpendicular to the fulcrum. If the eye level is not even with the fulcrum level, the wrong level may be set.

It is important that the researcher place the exposed films in order (e.g., one on top of another). Thus, when the films are processed, they are easily identified relative to the respective tomographic level.

CONCLUSION

In evaluating the tomograms, the researcher should be able to determine if the level set is the level obtained. For example, if a 5-cm level was set, but the number 6 was clear on the tomogram, there is something wrong. The experimenter should be able to determine what was wrong. In this case, some problems may be: experimenter's eye level was not perpendicular to the fulcrum level resulting in the wrong level being set, the number in the block doesn't coincide with the fulcrum level set, the tomographic unit is not operating properly.

A second, and related, conclusion the experimenter should address is that the tomogram is clearest at the fulcrum level. The concept of image thickness should not be mentioned as the exposure angle was constant, therefore, the thickness was the same.

ANSWERS TO QUESTIONS

1. Why are structures located at the fulcrum level well defined on a tomogram?

   The image of the anatomical section of interest (fulcrum level) stays in the same position on the film throughout the course of the tube movement and hence is clearly defined.

2. How should the areas above and below the fulcrum level appear on a tomogram?

   Images of structures which lie in planes above or below the plane of interest move at a different rate of speed than the film. In these cases, the image is obscured (blurred) in the resulting tomogram because they have moved across the film during the exposure.

3. What is the effect of changing the fulcrum level in conventional tomography?

   The fulcrum is variable and may be set at the level of the anatomical section (plane) of interest. The result is a clear image at the fulcrum level.

4. List 2 methods used to change the fulcrum level.

   Two methods used to adjust the fulcrum level are adjusting the fulcrum point of the bar that connects the x-ray tube and bucky tray (moveable fulcrum) and adjusting the bucky to accommodate a fixed fulcrum point.

TOMOGRAPHY: EFFECT OF EXPOSURE ANGLE ON THICKNESS OF OBJECTIVE PLANE

Some tomographic units use amplitude charts. On these units, the thickness may be influenced by the source image distance, rate of tube movement, etc. Thus, employing these types of units for this laboratory is discouraged. A tomographic unit with the capability to change the exposure angle is recommended.

EQUIPMENT

It is best to use a wire mesh block or other instrument which contains numbers (in centimeter increments) for measuring the thickness of the plane. The type of tomographic movement, e.g., linear, circular, influences the thickness of the objective plane. Thus, the more precise the unit, the need to employ a wire mesh block with precise measurements increases, e.g., millimeter.

CONCLUSION

The larger the exposure angle, the thinner the objective plane.

ANSWERS TO QUESTIONS

1. Define "exposure angle."

   The exposure angle in tomography (measured in angular degrees) is the angle formed at the fulcrum by the central ray during the travel of the tube over the course of the exposure.

2. What effect does increasing the exposure angle have on the thickness of the objective plane?

   The larger the exposure angle used to make a tomogram, the thinner the well-resolved (clearly defined) section (slice) in the resulting tomogram.

3. When would it be best to use a large exposure angle?

   It is best to use a large exposure angle when tomographing organs that are small organs, e.g., inner ear.

4. When would it be best to use a small exposure angle?

   It is best to use a small exposure angle when tomographing organs that are large, e.g., lungs, kidneys.

27

PROCESSING

AREA DESIGN

Most schools have 1 processing area. This often results in the processing area becoming crowded during the performance of this laboratory. To reduce the crowding, the students can be divided into 3 groups. All groups perform different aspects of the laboratory simultaneously. For example, one group can perform the observations of the viewing section of the processing area (procedural steps 1 and 2), another group of students does the observations of the developing area entrance (procedural steps 3 and 4) and the last group of students performs the observations of the developing area (procedural steps 5 and 6).

PROCEDURE

The procedure is designed to provide the student the opportunity to learn about processing area design by practical experience. Often students are overly concerned about how well they are able to draw diagrams of the area and equipment. This concern tends to overshadow the objective of the laboratory. To alleviate the students' concern over art work, the instructor should emphasize that their art quality is not a factor in grading. The students should be encouraged to draw "sketches" of the area and "major" equipment rather than concentrating on the details of the objects.

Since the visual appearance of the art may subconsciously influence the instructor's opinion of the quality of the laboratory, it is suggested that the instructor make a list of the items and diagram labeling needed for each observation section of the experiment. The list can be correlated with the respective observation section to assess the student's ability to identify important items.

OBSERVATION SECTIONS

In each respective observation section, the student draws a sketch of the respective area. The sketches should include the design of the area and items of major importance. The items in the sketch should be labeled appropriately. The items to be included in the sketches vary according to each respective school's processing area design. Also, as mentioned previously, the instructor should encourage the student to concentrate on sketching the important items rather than the small details and art quality.

CONCLUSION

The conclusion should reflect a written summary of the design of the viewing section, developing area entrance and developing area design. The summary should contain information about the type of design, e.g., double door entrance, and type of equipment located in each section.

This experiment is written to familiarize the student with the processing area. The uses of the various equipment are not a part of this experiment. Instructors wishing to have the student include the uses of the various equipment items should advise the student ahead of time and have the student edit the laboratory accordingly.

ANSWERS TO QUESTIONS

1. What are the two primary sections of a processing area?

   The two primary sections of the processing area are the viewing section and developing section.

2. What is the purpose of the developing section?

   The developing section is where film is loaded, unloaded and fed into the processor for processing.

3. What is the purpose of the viewing area?

   The viewing section is where the "dry" radiograph is viewed.

4. Identify three different types of entrances that may be used to enter the developing section of the processing area?

   The 3 types of entrances are single door, double door and revolving door.

5. Where is the automatic (or manual) processor located?

   The automatic processor extends through the wall dividing the viewing and developing sections. Thus, part of the processor is located in the developing section and part is in the viewing section.

28

PROCESSING

AREA

QUALITY

CONTROL

PROCEDURE

Students sometimes have difficulty determining if an item is pass or fail. The researcher should be encouraged to fail anything that does not meet the standard by 100%.

Instructors may elect to use a safelight test other than the one listed in the laboratory. If this is the case, the instructor needs to provide the student with the necessary information to complete the test. Instructors using the test in the laboratory are advised that the timing of the safelight exposure and moving of the paper down the film is difficult when performed in the dark. One way to facilitate timing is to use a timer which can easily be set for 30 seconds and sounds a bell when the time has expired. To assist in moving the film by 1 inch lengths, the side of the paper used to shield the 1/4 edge of the film may be marked with masking tape at 1 inch intervals. Care needs to be taken to avoid placing tape on a cardboard holder such that it tears the holder when it is removed.

DATA

All areas must be checked as either pass or fail. Those checked as fail must have a statement in the comment section to explain why the test failed. The results are dependent upon the types of problems that may exist in the respective researcher's processing area.

S U M M A R Y   O F   F I N D I N G S

Students often confuse the content of the Summary of findings and Recommendation sections. This section contains information which outlines the findings listed in the data section. For example, there is a crack in the safelight filter. Specific findings depend upon the processing area efficiency.

R E C O M M E N D A T I O N S   A N D   C O N C L U S I O N

This section is closely related to the Summary of findings. It contains information as to what to do or how to fix the items which failed the tests. Continuing with the Summary of findings example, the recommendation is to replace the filter with a new one. All recommendations should represent permanent solutions. For example, if a researcher said to tape the crack in the filter, the answer is incorrect.

The conclusion can be a general statement about the status of the processing area. For example, the processing area was found to be in good order with only a few deficiencies.

The specific recommendations and conclusion are dependant upon the results in the data.

ANSWERS TO QUESTIONS

1. List 2 reasons why repeat radiographs are undesirable.

    Repeat radiographs are undesirable because they increase radiation exposure to the patient and increase costs to the radiography department.

2. List 2 things that individuals may do to avoid foreign substances from contaminating the processing area.

    To avoid foreign substances from entering either the chemicals or film holders, individuals should refrain from eating, smoking or drinking in the processing area.

3. Identify 2 areas where white light leaks are commonly found in a processing area.

    Common areas where white leaks are usually located include between the processor and wall, under doors and where pipes enter the developing section.

4. Why shouldn't films be stacked on top of one another when they are stored?

    Stacking film may cause artifacts in the form of pressure marks on the film.

29

PROCESSOR PARTS AND FUNCTION

EQUIPMENT

One of the 3 experiments requires the researcher to remove racks from the processor. Since the deep racks are in solution, a towel should be used to absorb any excess liquid from the rollers.

EXPERIMENT 1

PROCEDURE

The instructor is advised that soft contact lenses absorb moisture. Therefore, care should be taken to ensure that individuals wearing soft contact lenses avoid getting near solutions, especially the fixer, since the vapors may be absorbed by the contact lenses.

When removing the deep rack, there is a potential for the solution of one tank to "drip" into another, e.g., the developer may fall into the fixer. The individual(s) removing the rack should use the towels to catch any excess solution to avoid cross contamination.

When diagraming the racks, it is not unusual for students to be overly concerned about their art work rather than identifying the appropriate items on the rack. Instructors should encourage the researcher to concentrate on the contents of the rack and reinforce that art is not a part of the grade.

VISUAL OBSERVATION

The researcher should diagram each rack. It is recommended that the student use the manual provided by the manufacturing company to determine the names of the rack parts.

Using the manual enables the student to label the correct parts and familiarizes the researcher with the type of information provided with the processor. The specific items identified depend on the type of processor.

CONCLUSION

This section should contain information comparing and contrasting the racks. For example, all racks contain guide shoes, but only the deep rack has a large turnaround roller. This laboratory does not address the difference between a face to face or zigzag roller configuration. Instructors wishing to include that in the experiment are encouraged to advise the student of the requirement.

EXPERIMENT 2

PROCEDURE

The instructor is advised that soft contact lenses absorb moisture. Therefore, care should be taken to ensure that individuals wearing soft contact lenses avoid getting near solutions, especially the fixer, since the vapors may be absorbed by the contact lenses.

The developer and fixer tanks have a small amount of space between the racks and solutions. The film should be place in the space and agitated. After the film has been submerged in both tanks, it is suggested the ends be placed in the wash to remove any fixer or developer solutions. The processor may then be turned on and allowed to warm up. Once the dryer reaches the proper temperature, the film may be placed in the dryer to dry. The film should be attached to the laboratory report as data.

VISUAL OBSERVATION

Students often write the conclusion in this section. To avoid this from happening, the instructor should emphasize the importance of writing only what is visible. Thus, the researcher would be able to conclude that the film turned black when submerged in the developer and was clear when submerged in the fixer.

CONCLUSION

The developer turned the exposed crystals to metallic silver. The fixer removed all crystals, exposed and unexposed.

EXPERIMENT 3

VISUAL OBSERVATION

As in experiment number 2, this section often reflects the conclusion. It should contain a summary of what was seen. The type of information included here is direction of film movement, e.g., entrance rack to developer, color of film as it passed from rack to rack, bell sounded when film entered processor, replenishment system starts, etc.

CONCLUSION

As the film enters the processor, it activates a switch which starts the replenishment system. After it completely entered the developer tank, a bell sounded signaling that it is okay to enter another film. The film travels through the processor from the developer, fixer, wash and dryer. In the developer, the ionized crystals are changed to metallic silver. The fixer removed all unexposed crystals. The wash removed any solution residue and the dryer dried the film. The time to process the film was about 90 seconds.

ANSWERS TO QUESTIONS

1. List 2 functions of the entrance rack.

   The entrance rack picks up the film from the tray and transports it to the developer. During this process, a detector system is energized. The detector system warns the user if 2 films are overlapped by sounding a buzzer, tells the user when the film is in the developer by sounding a bell and activates the replenishment system.

2. What function does the developer serve?

   The function of the developer is to change the ionized crystals (latent image) to metallic silver (manifest image).

3. What is the function of the D-F cross-over rack?

   The developer-fixer (D-F) cross-over rack transports the film from the developer to the fixer tank. This rack also removes excess developer, preventing contamination of the fixer.

4. What function does the fixer serve?

   The fixer removes any remaining silver bromide crystals (clears the film).

30

PROCESSOR
INSPECTION

The potential problems associated with this laboratory are very similar to the Processing area quality control and Processor parts and function laboratories. For example, students sometimes have difficulty determining if an item is pass or fail. The researcher should be encouraged to fail anything that does not meet the standard by 100%. As always, the instructor is advised that soft contact lens absorb moisture. Therefore, care should be taken to ensure that individuals wearing soft contact lens avoid getting near solutions, especially the fixer, since the vapors may be absorbed by the contact lens.

When removing the deep rack, there is a potential for the solution of one tank to "drip" into another, e.g., the developer may fall into the fixer. The individual(s) removing the rack should use the towels to catch any excess solution to avoid cross contamination. The racks should be placed on a table or counter which is large enough to accommodate all the racks.

EXPERIMENT 1

PROCEDURE

To ensure the film hits the entrance roller and is lifted off the feed tray, the researcher should have their eye level even with the film and entrance roller. Also, the white lights of the developing section should be on.

When removing the deep racks, it is important to avoid cross contamination of the developer and fixer. Consequently, the racks should be removed slowly. A splash guard and towel may be used to absorb excess solution.

EXPERIMENT 2

PROCEDURE

To visualize if the solutions are circulating, all tanks must be filled with the respective solutions (including the water tank) and all racks must be out of the processor.

It is important that the processor be off when inspecting the filter. If the processor is on, developer solution may spill out of the filter casing.

EXPERIMENT 4

PROCEDURE

When checking the temperature of the dryer, avoid using a mercury thermometer. Employing mercury thermometers may result in mercury spilling if the thermometer is accidently broken.

DATA

All areas must be checked as either pass or fail. Those checked as fail must have a statement in the comment section to explain why the test failed. The results are dependent upon the types of problems that may exist in the respective researcher's processor.

SUMMARY OF FINDINGS

Students often confuse the content of the Summary of findings and Recommendation sections. This section contains information which outlines the findings listed in the data section. For example, there is a crack in a gear on a transportation roller. Specific findings depend upon the processor status.

RECOMMENDATIONS AND CONCLUSION

This section is closely related to the summary of findings. It contains information as to what to do or how to fix the items which failed the tests. Continuing with the Summary of findings example, the recommendation is to replace the roller with a new one. All recommendations should represent permanent solutions.

The conclusion can be a general statement about the status of the processor. For example, the processor was found to be in good order with only a few deficiencies.

The specific recommendations and conclusion are dependent upon the results in the data.

ANSWERS TO QUESTIONS

1. How often should the parts of an automatic processor be inspected?

    The frequency of part inspection depends on the durability of the part. Some parts wear away faster than others and are inspected daily. Other parts are more durable and inspection occurs at longer time intervals, e.g., weekly or monthly.

2. What is the function of the transportation system?

    The transportation system moves the film through the developer, fixer, wash and dryer at the correct speed without damaging the film.

3. List 3 items on a rack that should be inspected:

    The following are potential answers to question 3

    a. rollers are in good condition (no damage or dirt).

    b. guide shoes (deflector plates) are aligned properly. The entrance of the guide shoe is wide to catch the film and the exit is narrow.

    c. gears are in good condition (no cracks or missing teeth) and aligned.

    d. the detector arm turns on the detector switch when a film passes through the entrance rack.

    e. since crossover and the squeegee racks are out of water, check to ensure the rollers are not dried out.

    f. the deep rack chains are adjusted properly and are tightened appropriately.

    g. check gears of racks to ensure they are operating properly.

    h. dryer belt on the blower is of proper tension.

4. Why would the tube of the replenishment system be checked for kinks, cracks or debris?

    The tubing is inspected for kinks, cracks, leaks or any obstruction which may hinder the flow of chemicals.

5. What "causes" hot air to be circulated in the dryer?

    The blower circulates the hot air in the dryer.

31

SUBTRACTION

This experiment demonstrates only first order subtraction. If the instructor wishes to demonstrate second or third order subtraction as well, it is recommended that the instructor refer to the text *Fundamentals of Angiography* by Dr. Marianne Tortorici.

EQUIPMENT

The expense of subtraction machines and automatic processors limits the quantity of this type of equipment available in the majority of schools to 1 or 2. Therefore, this laboratory is best performed in small groups rather than individually. Each group should be assigned to the developing side of the processing area one at a time. This requires the groups to work in "shifts."

PROCEDURE

Exposing the film by the white light method versus using a subtraction machine introduces subjectivity and the possibility of error into the timing of the exposure. Two or more films may have to be exposed before an appropriate exposure time can be established.

In the case of exposing the film without a subtraction machine, it is suggested that the individuals in each group be assigned specific tasks to avoid confusion. For example, one person controls placing the film under the white light source and a second person controls the light exposure. When the film is properly positioned, the "film person" tells the "light person" to make the exposure. For the sake of consistency, the person who made the first light exposure should also make the repeat exposure(s) in a situation where an exposure needs to be repeated.

Subtraction film has emulsion on only one side. The emulsion side of the subtraction film must be facing the film(s) to be subtracted and the white light source for the film to perform its function. Subtraction film has a notched corner to indicate which side of the film contains the emulsion; if the notch is placed in either the lower right hand corner or the upper left hand corner, the emulsion side is facing up. Also, subtraction film has a shiny side and a dull side; the dull side is the emulsion side. Thus, the subtraction film should be positioned with the dull side facing the light source.

VISUAL OBSERVATION

Base—the experimenter should describe the objects visualized on the radiograph relative to black and white shades.

Mask—the experimenter should record that the image densities on the mask are the reverse of the base film.

Contrast film—this film should demonstrate what additional objects were added to the base film.

Print—this should demonstrate the objects added to the contrast film. The objects of the base film should be barely visible. Often the original objects have some visibility on the film. If a great deal of the original objects can be seen, it is possible the mask was not dark enough and should be repeated.

CONCLUSION

Subtraction is a photographic method used to demonstrate objects that may be obscured by other anatomical parts.

ANSWERS TO QUESTIONS

1. What is the purpose of radiographic subtraction?

   Subtraction is a technique whereby unwanted detail can be subtracted from radiographs leaving the desired detail visible.

2. Subtraction is used mainly in what field of radiography?

   Subtraction is most commonly used in angiographic procedures.

3. What purpose does the mask film serve?

   The mask is an exact negative of everything in the contrast film but the objects containing the radiopaque material. When combined with the contrast film the images cancel each other out (whatever is light in one is equally dark in the other) everywhere except the objects containing the radiopaque material.

32

STEREO-
RADIOGRAPHY

PROCEDURE

It is essential that the radiographs be placed correctly on the illuminator. The films are placed on the illuminator in the same position as if seen by the tube, the left stereoradiograph on the viewer's left and the right on the viewer's right with the tube side of the film facing the observer. If the student can't see 3-D, it is possible the films are on the wrong view box or may need to be "flipped" over (rotated on their vertical axis).

The authors have run into 2 additional problems with viewing the radiographs. One problem results when the interpupillary distance of the viewer is not 2.5 inches. In these cases, the films can be repeated changing the ratio to match the ratio of the student's interpupillary distance with the 25-inch view distance. For example a 2.2-inch distance results in a 2.2/25 ratio or a 0.09 % tube shift. For a 40 SID the total shift would be 3.6 inches (0.09 x 40 = 3.6). The second problem is that not everyone has the ability to see depth. It has been the authors' experience that these individuals were unaware that they could not see depth. After the inability to see the films in 3-D, several researchers went to an optometrist or ophthalmologist and discovered they had no depth perception. Consequently, the instructor is advised to be aware that students who indicate that they cannot see 3-D may be unable to see depth.

For this experiment, the anatomical part selected should have enough complexity to see depth, e.g., skull. Also, the radiographs must be taken bucky even if the part does not normally require a bucky technique. This is because table top radiographs require the object to be moved. In stereoradiography, the object must remain in the same position.

The direction of tube movement is critical. Moving the tube to be perpendicular to the lead strips of the grid causes grid cut off. Thus, the object must be placed on the table so the longitudinal axis of the part will result in the tube movement being parallel to the longitudinal axis of the lead strips.

In step 7, the total distance the tube moves is 4 inches. This results in the tube being 2 inches to the opposite side of the center of the object.

VISUAL OBSERVATION

The radiographs viewed separately demonstrate length and width (2 dimensions). When viewed with a stereo viewer, the added dimension of depth was visible.

CONCLUSION

It is possible to demonstrate depth using a special radiographic technique called stereoradiography.

ANSWERS TO QUESTIONS

1. Define stereoradiography.

   Stereoradiography is a radiographic technique used to demonstrate depth.

2. What is the total tube shift of a stereoradiograph taken at 72 inch SID (show math)?

   The total tube shift is 7.2 inches or 0.10 x 72 = 7.2 inches.

3. Name 2 methods of viewing stereoradiographs.

   There are several ways to view stereoradiographs, including direct vision, stereomonoculars, stereobinoculars and more sophisticated stereoscopes.

4. If a 3-D object cannot be viewed when looking at stereoradiographs, list 2 things that might be wrong.

   The radiographs may need to be turned on their vertical axis, or their location on the illuminator switched. The interpupillary distance of the viewer may not be 2.5 inches. The individual may not be able to see depth.

33

FILM

DUPLICATION

PROCEDURE

Common errors made by the student are not locking the lid and using the wrong compensation time, if needed. The instructor is encouraged to advise the researcher of the importance of locking the top of the duplicating machine. Failure to do so will result in a blurry copy. Since the manner in which to obtain a lighter or darker copy is the reverse of conventional radiography, it is recommended that the instructor emphasize the importance of how to compensate for copies that are too light or too dark.

VISUAL OBSERVATION

The researcher should record the fact that the copy is the same as the original. The primary difference between the 2 is that the duplicating film is "shiny" (this is because the film is single emulsion). If the copy was too light or dark and needed repeating, it should be recorded in this section.

CONCLUSION

It is possible to copy a radiograph such that the image produced is the same as the original radiograph.

ANSWERS TO QUESTIONS

1. List 2 reasons for duplicating radiographs.

   Some uses of film duplication are mailing radiographs, providing physicians with copies of their patient's examination or using radiographs for teaching purposes.

2. When duplicating a radiograph, what is the correct order to place the radiograph and duplication film relative to the light source?

The emulsion side of the duplication film must be in close contact with the radiograph to be copied and the light source must be facing the original radiograph and emulsion side of the duplicating film.

3. If a film duplicated using a 4-second exposure is too dark, what should be done to lighten the film?

The exposure time should be increased.

34

SENSITOMETRY

INTRODUCTION

This laboratory defines sensitometry as being performed daily. However, most educational systems are not designed to provide the student the opportunity to perform daily sensitometry readings. Therefore, this laboratory is written to allow the experimenter the opportunity to perform sensitometry in 3 consecutive laboratories or class periods. Instructors may wish to increase the number of times the researcher performs sensitometry. The more measurements the experimenter records, the more accurate the results.

Often radiographic laboratories are used by several different classes. Thus, a need exists to ensure the control film box is used only by those performing the sensitometry tests. If the control box becomes empty, a cross over must be performed. The introduction section of the laboratory contains information on how to perform a cross over.

Since the density is processor dependent, the instructor should make sure the processor is warmed up prior to use. Also, it is recommended that several large scrap films be "run" through the processor before developing the sensitometry strip.

EXPERIMENT 1

CONCLUSION

The standard temperature for the processor varies according to the type of processor employed. The researcher should be able to record the proper temperature and the acceptable range. The instructor may wish to have a copy of the processor manual on hand for the experimenters to review relative to the manufacturer's recommended temperature.

EXPERIMENT 2

FILM EXPOSURE

Instructors should make sure the experimenters use the appropriate color sensitivity setting when exposing the film to the sensitometer. Also, the experimenter may wish to look at the sensitometer film strip (the one located on the sensitometer) to determine where the dark steps are located. This will enable the researcher to determine which end of the test film will have the lightest density. Knowing the end with the lightest density helps in properly inserting the film in the processor.

Double emulsion film seems to present the greatest problem with this experiment. Both emulsions must be exposed. To ensure the same respective emulsion is being obtained from one day to the next, it is recommended that special care be taken to lift the film from the box in the same manner. When the film is removed from the box, the researcher can label the film in one corner for identification upon development. Also, to expose both emulsions, the film must be "flipped over." Rotating the film 180 degrees while it is in the same plane exposes the opposite side of the SAME emulsion.

CONCLUSION

The density standards vary according to the type of film and processing conditions. The student should be able to identify the standards and their acceptable ranges in this section.

EXPERIMENT 3

CONCLUSION

The results are dependent upon the function of the processor. In general, the researcher should be able to identify unacceptable readings and possible problems creating the variance. Also, if a significant number of tests were performed, the experimenter should be able to identify when a trend, e.g., density began increasing, started. It is also important for the researcher to note if the processor is performing properly.

ANSWERS TO QUESTIONS

1. Define sensitometry

   Sensitometry is a method used to study and measure the relationship of exposure, processing conditions and film response.

2. What types of densities are recorded in sensitometry? How often are they recorded?

   Film fog, speed and contrast are the densities recorded in sensitometry. These readings are taken daily.

3. What is the advantage of implementing a sensitometry program?

   The objective of sensitometry is to ensure the processor is operating at a consistent and acceptable level.

4. What are the generally accepted limits for film fog, speed, contrast and chemical temperature?

   The acceptable limit for film fog is ± 0.02. The acceptable limit for speed and contrast is ± 0.10. The chemical temperature limit is ± 1 degree.

35

SILVER RECOVERY

RECOMMENDATIONS AND CONCLUSION BASED ON THE DATA

The experimenter must identify the type of silver recovery system for the processor and its security system. The researcher must also identify the manner in which the discarded films are stored and the security system. If there is no silver recovery system or there is a problem with the system/security, the researcher must list recommendations to correct the errors.

ANSWERS TO QUESTIONS

1. List two methods used to recover silver from the fixer.

   There are two methods used to collect silver from the fixer. They are the metallic replacement (cartridge) and electrolytic methods.

2. Approximately how many troy ounces can be recovered from 1 gallon of fixer?

   Approximately 0.5 to 0.8 troy ounces may be recovered per gallon of fixer.

3. If the average troy ounce yield for 1,000 sheets of 10" x 12" film is 11.1, what is the mean (average) troy ounces that can be expected from 16,000 sheets of 10" x 12" film. (Show math.)

$$16,000/1,000 = 16$$

$$16 \times 11.1 = 177.6 \text{ troy ounces}$$

4. If silver is selling at $ 6.25/troy ounce, how much money should be expected from question #3? (Show math.)

$$177.6 \times \$ 6.25 = \$ 1,110.00$$

5. List 3 types of discarded film.

   Three types of discarded film are Green, Archival and Reject film.

6. What type of discarded film has the highest silver content?

   Green films contain the greatest amount of silver.

36

INTENSIFYING SCREEN LIGHT EMISSION

EQUIPMENT

Some departments have only 1 type of intensifying screen. Although this laboratory is designed to demonstrate blue and green light emission, it may still be employed for departments with only 1 screen type available.

PROCEDURE

When the room lights are turned off, the room becomes very dark and presents safety hazards. If view boxes are unavailable, a need exists to establish some form of dim lighting, e.g., small incandescent light. Avoid leaving the x-ray room door ajar to have hallway light enter the x-ray room as this is against proper radiation protection practices. If no form of illumination is available, some procedure should be established to perform the experiment while maintaining proper safety methods.

It is recommended that the instructor employ several different cassettes for the laboratory even if the intensifying screens emit the same color light.

VISUAL OBSERVATION

The experimenter should be able to properly identify the color of light emitted and if there was any screen lag for all cassettes.

CONCLUSION

Intensifying screens emit a light when irradiated. The color of the light depends upon the type of intensifying screen. No light is emitted after the exposure ended (if the researcher experienced some afterglow he/she should comment on the effects and recommendations regarding the screen lag). The experimenter should specifically identify the type of screens he/she employed and the light color emitted.

ANSWERS TO QUESTIONS

1. What is the purpose of an intensifying screen?

   Intensifying screens significantly decrease the amount of radiation needed to produce a radiographic image, providing the opportunity to image large organs.

2. What is the difference between fluorescence and phosphorescence?

   Fluorescence emits light only when stimulated. Phosphorescence continues to emit light after the stimulation has stopped.

3. What is spectrum matching?

   Correlating the color of the screen with the film is termed "spectrum matching."

4. What is the difference between panchromatic and orthochromatic film?

   Panchromatic film is manufactured to be blue-violet light sensitive while orthochromatic is green light sensitive.

INTENSIFYING SCREEN RESOLUTION

EQUIPMENT

It may be difficult to locate a resolution grid that can measure 120 lp/mm. It is recommended to use the highest possible lp/mm grid available.

It is also recommended that the instructor use screens with a large variance in speed, e.g., extremity cassette.

PROCEDURE

Make sure the experimenter obtains a film with a density of about 1.2. If the radiograph is too light or too dark, it presents difficulties in reading the lp/mm.

If using a resolution grid that has a minimum of 5 lp/mm, it may not be sensitive enough to measure the resolution of fast screens. It is more common to have a grid that is not sensitive enough (not enough lp/mm) to demonstrate the resolution of the cardboard film holder. In both these cases, the experimenter can only conclude that the resolution could not be determined. In the former case, the researcher can only conclude that the resolution is somewhere below 5 lp/mm and in the latter instance, the resolution is somewhere above the "x" lp/mm grid used.

DATA

The experimenter should be able to identify the resolution level for all film holders. As mentioned in the procedure section, if all lp/mm are blurred, the researcher must state that he/she was unable to determine the resolution level, but it is above or below "x" lp/mm (depending upon the image). See procedure section.

CONCLUSION

The experimenter should be able to identify the rank order of resolution for the film holders tested.

ANSWERS TO QUESTIONS

1. What tool is used to measure intensifying screen resolution?

   A resolution grid is used to measure intensifying screen resolution.

2. How many lead strips and gaps are in 10 lp/mm resolution grid?

   There are 10 lead lines and gaps in a 10 lp/mm resolution grid.

3. If cassette A resolves 8 lp/mm and cassette B resolves 5 lp/mm, which cassette provides the clearer image and why?

   Cassette A will be clearer because it is able to resolve more lp/mm.

4. List 3 factors that influence image sharpness relative to intensifying screens.

   Among the primary factors influencing image sharpness resulting from intensifying screens are

   a. screen speed

   b. cross-over

   c. screen contact

   d. quantum mottle

5. What effect does divergent light rays have on image quality?

   Divergent rays cause an increase in penumbra decreasing image quality.

38

INTENSIFYING SCREEN CONTACT

MATERIAL

It is important that the wire mesh be completely flat. Any warping of the wire mesh causes an object film distance which may be interpreted as poor screen contact.

Also, the object placed in the cassette must be soft to prevent damaging the screens. The object must be of sufficient size to create poor screen contact. Avoid large objects as they can damage the cassette. Do not continue to close the cassette if a significant resistance is met when locking the cassette.

OBSERVATION

The normal radiograph demonstrates excellent radiographic quality all over the film. It has high contrast and the wire mesh lines are sharp. The radiograph labeled "object" demonstrates good screen contact where the object is pressing the film against the screen, but there are blurring and an increase in density around the object.

CONCLUSION

Sometimes the experimenter tends to summarize the experiment by stating that in order to create poor screen contact put an object in the cassette. The instructor should stress that placing an object in the cassette is intended to simulate the effect of poor screen contact and is not performed as a routine practice.

The researcher should conclude that the optimum radiographic quality is obtained when there is good screen film contact. If there is a question of poor screen contact, a wire mesh test may be performed.

ANSWERS TO QUESTIONS

1. What effect does poor screen contact have on radiographic quality and why?

   Failure of intensifying screens to make good contact with the film results in the divergence of the light emitted from the screen during exposure. This light divergence causes blurring (penumbra) that obscures small detail creating a loss of contrast and radiographic quality.

2. List 2 causes of poor screen contact.

   Any damage to the screen or foreign objects may cause poor screen contact.

3. How can poor screen contact be avoided?

   Poor screen contact may be avoided by handling the screen carefully to prevent damage and cleaning the cassettes on a regular basis.

GRID LINES

VISUAL OBSERVATION

The first 2 radiographs demonstrate grid lines. The width of the grid's lead strips determines whether or not the lines hinder the image. Many modern grids have very thin lead strips making the effect of the lines on the image negligible. The last radiograph, number 3, has the lead strips of the grid moving, thus, there is no image of the lead on the radiograph. This improves the radiographic quality of the image.

CONCLUSION

Grids are useful in removing the secondary and scatter radiation. However, if a stationary grid is employed, the lead strips appear on the radiograph as grid lines. Although the lead is visible on the radiograph, the improved quality of the film justifies using the stationary grid. If a grid is needed, it is best to employ a moving grid to obtain an optimum radiograph.

ANSWERS TO QUESTIONS

1. Define grid.

   Grids used in radiography consist of an arrangement of alternating lead and radiolucent strips through which most of the primary x-ray photons pass to reach the x-ray film.

2. List 2 causes of grid lines when using a bucky.

   Using a stationary grid and a bucky which is out of sequence will cause grid lines.

3. When should a grid be used in radiography?

   Grids should be used for parts measuring 6 inches (15 cm) or greater and containing fairly dense tissue.

4. What is the advantage of using a grid?

   The lead strips of the grid intercept many of the scattered primary photons and secondary photons which result from interactions with the air, tissue and equipment. Reduction of the number of scattered and secondary photons reaching the film reduces the blurring or "fog" in the radiographic image.

5. What is a disadvantage of using a stationary grid?

   The disadvantage of a stationary grid is that it causes grid lines on the radiograph.

40

GRID CUT OFF

EQUIPMENT

The equipment list identifies a 10:1 grid be used for this experiment. Any grid ratio is capable of demonstrating the causes of grid cut off. Although the grid ratio is not an important factor in this experiment, the use of a stationary grid is relevant. The stationary grid provides the flexibility to place the grid in various positions enabling the demonstration of all causes of grid cut off. Employing a moving grid (Potter-Bucky type) for this laboratory limits the number of causes which can be demonstrated. Besides grid type, knowing the manner in which the grid is constructed and having labels on the grid are important.

Some grids are constructed so the length of the lead strips run the length of the grid while other grids have the lead strip length positioned to extend the width of the grid. The manner is which the lead is positioned in the grid does not affect the experiment. However, it is vital that the user know which way the lead is placed in the grid. Knowing the lead strip position in the grid enables the experimenter to angle the tube relative to the strips. For example, if the lead strips are lengthwise, then to demonstrate grid cut off, the tube angle must be in the direction of the width of the grid. Angling the tube to coincide with the lengthwise position of the grid causes the x-ray beam to be parallel to the lead and does not demonstrate grid cut off.

The last important item is to ensure the grid contains a legible label. The label should include grid ratio, type of grid (parallel or focused), focal range, etc.

PROCEDURE

Care needs to be taken to ensure that students position the tube and grid to demonstrate grid cut off. As previously mentioned, the experimenter must be aware of the position of the lead strips in the grid. To demonstrate grid cut off by incorrect beam angle, the tube must be angled perpendicular to the lead strips. Also, the decentering portion of the laboratory requires the tube to be moved so that if a line was drawn from where the central ray (CR) meets the grid to the center lead strip of the grid, the line would be perpendicular to the long axis (length) of the lead strips.

The focal range part of the experiment is best demonstrated by placing the tube at a distance which is significantly greater than the recommended focal range. This exaggerates the grid cut off effect making it readily visible on the radiograph. Care needs to be taken to adjust the radiographic technique to obtain a diagnostic film.

This laboratory has the experimenter demonstrate grid cut off by incorrect angle of the x-ray beam and employing an angled grid. In both these procedures, the angle employed is critical. It is recommended that an angle no greater than 5 degrees be employed. Angles greater than 5 degrees create too much grid cut off resulting in a clear radiograph.

As mentioned earlier, it is important to use a focused grid. This is critical when attempting to demonstrate the effect of an inverted grid. Employing a parallel grid for the inverted focused grid procedure does not demonstrate grid cut off.

VISUAL OBSERVATIONS

In this section, the experimenter should list the visual effects demonstrated on each radiograph. It is recommended that this be expressed in terms of the photographic image quality. Also, the experimenter may wish to identify the area of the film demonstrating the grid cut off. For example, in the inverted focused grid portion, the grid cut off is seen on the lateral sides of the image (assuming the lead strips are lengthwise and the phantom part is positioned lengthwise on the film).

Besides grid cut off, grid lines are visualized on the radiograph. The importance of having the experimenter identify the grid lines is at the discretion of the instructor. There is a separate experiment on grid lines which is better used to illustrate grid lines.

CONCLUSION

This section should contain information relative to the causes of grid cut off. It is also recommended that the experimenter identify grid cut off as being undesirable. However, students tend to be so concerned about listing all the types of grid cut off, they sometimes forget to mention that grid cut off is undesirable. Thus, it is recommended that the instructor advise the students that the conclusion contain information about the causes and effect of grid cut off.

ANSWERS TO QUESTIONS

1. Define grid.

   Grids used in radiography consist of an alternate arrangement of lead strips and radiolucent material through which most of the primary photons pass.

2. What is the function of a grid?

   The function of a grid is to reduce the number of scattered photons reaching the film, blurring or "fogging" the radiographic image.

3. Define grid cut off.

   The unwanted absorption of the primary x-ray beam by a grid is called grid cut off.

4. List at least 3 ways of obtaining grid cut off.

   The following is a list of the ways of obtaining grid cut off.

   a. tube focus is outside the focal range

   b. improper tube angulation

   c. unlevel grid

   d. inverted focused grid

   e. lateral decentering

41

BEAM RESTRICTORS: X-RAY BEAM AND LIGHT ACCURACY

There are 3 quality control tests in this laboratory. They are tests for

1. x-ray beam light projected relative to the irradiated field.

2. location of the center of the irradiated field relative to the center of the film.

3. angle of the central ray.

Students tend to have trouble discriminating between tests 1 and 2 above. They often see them as being one test. Thus, the instructor is advised to emphasize the differences among the various tests.

PROCEDURE

The instructor should check to make sure the cassette is centered in the bucky tray. If the cassette is off centered, it will cause erroneous test results.

CONCLUSION

The conclusion depends upon how accurate the collimator light corresponds to the radiation. The results are also influenced by the accuracy of the central ray angle. It is suggested the instructor review the radiographs for possible collimator light or central ray misalignment. The student's conclusion should reflect the level of accuracy of the equipment.

ANSWERS TO QUESTIONS

1. Why is it important for the collimator light to represent the irradiated field?

   Misalignment of the collimator light and radiation may result in repeating the radiograph. This increases the radiation absorption to the patient.

2. What may cause misalignment of the collimator light?

   Misalignment of the collimator light may be caused if the tube is hit or during maintenance/repair work on the x-ray tube, tube enclosure or collimator.

3. For a 45 inch (114 cm) SID, what is the maximum acceptable misalignment distance?

$$45 \times 0.02 = 0.90 \text{ inches}$$

or

$$114 \times 0.02 = 2.28 \text{ cm}$$

4. According to federal regulations, what is the acceptable central ray angle?

   Perpendicular (90 degrees) to the image receptor.

5. If a 40 inch (100 cm) SID is employed and the center of the irradiated field is 0.5 inches to the left of the center of the film, is it within legal limitations? Please explain your answer.

   Yes, because 0.5 inches represents 1.25% of the SID. For the example to be illegal, the distance would have to exceed the legal limit of 2% of the SID.

42

EFFECT OF DISTORTION ON RADIOGRAPHIC QUALITY

This laboratory is designed to demonstrate the effect of shape distortion on radiographic quality. The particular type of radiographic quality of interest is image sharpness and shape of the object (e.g., foreshortening, elongation). Other laboratory experiments demonstrate the effect of additional factors, e.g., magnification, on radiographic quality.

EQUIPMENT

To avoid an outside or external influence of factors on radiographic quality other than distortion, a cardboard film holder is used. This eliminates the effect of intensifying screens on radiographic quality.

PROCEDURE

Students perform the 3 ways of obtaining shape distortion: angling the part, angling the tube and angling the film. Of these methods, angling the film presents the greatest challenge to the student. Many students tend to read the instructions correctly, but perform the method incorrectly.

The main problem is that the students tend to use a sponge to angle the film 45 degrees as indicated by the procedural steps, but place the phantom part against the film so the part is also angled 45 degrees. The instructor is encouraged to advise the student that the phantom part must be perpendicular to the central ray. Angling the part and film introduces 2 changes making it difficult for the experimenter to determine if the part, film or both created the resulting image.

CONCLUSION

The student should be able to identify the geometric distortion of the phantom part. In the angling of the tube, the part will be either elongated or foreshortened depending on whether the tube was angled caudal or cephalad relative to the position of the part. Angling the part 45 degrees tends to foreshorten the phantom part. Film angulation may elongate the portion of the part having the largest object film distance and foreshorten the portion closest to the film. The normal radiograph demonstrates an object of the same geometric shape, but may display magnification (size distortion). All distorted radiographs display penumbra in the form of image unsharpness.

ANSWERS TO QUESTIONS

1. Define distortion.

   Distortion is an uneven magnification of an object often seen as the geometric misrepresentation of an object (shape distortion).

2. What is the difference between size and shape distortion?

   In size distortion the object maintains the same geometric shape, but the size of the object is enlarged. Shape distortion results in the misrepresentation of the object's geometric pattern.

3. List three ways of obtaining shape distortion.

   Three ways of obtaining shape distortion are angling the part, angling the tube and angling the film.

4. Give an example of how distortion may be used to an advantage.

   This question has many answers. Any radiograph taken of an object in which the film and part are not perpendicular to the tube causes distortion. Examples include oblique views of a part and radiographs in which the tube is angled, e.g., posterior profile (Stenver's) projection of the skull.

43

EFFECT OF MAGNIFI-CATION ON RADIOGRAPHIC QUALITY

EQUIPMENT

It is important to use a flat object for the laboratory. A thick object creates magnification due to the varying OFDs within the object (e.g., the top of object has a different OFD than the bottom of the object).

Use nonscreen or other high resolution film holders to avoid introducing magnification due to the screens or other external factors. Also, the filming should be performed tabletop as bucky radiography introduces magnification.

A film large enough to have the entire object demonstrated on the radiograph should be employed. The actual size of the film needed will depend upon the size of the flat object employed.

EXPERIMENT 1

PROCEDURE

When decreasing the SID, it is important to remember to open the cones to irradiate the entire object.

DATA

Magnification for radiograph #1 is approximately 4.2%, radiograph #2 has a magnification of about 5.3% and the last radiograph's magnification is approximately 11.1%.

VISUAL OBSERVATION

As the SID decreased, the object increased in size and became blurry. Thus, the radiographic quality decreased.

CONCLUSION

The best radiographic quality is obtained with a small OFD to SOD ratio (OFD is small and SOD is large).

EXPERIMENT 2

DATA

The magnification for the first radiograph is 0, the second radiograph has a magnification of approximately 5.3% and the last radiograph's magnification is about 11.1%.

VISUAL OBSERVATION

As the OFD increased, the size of the object increased and the radiograph became blurry. Consequently, the radiographic quality decreased.

CONCLUSION

It is not unusual for students to compare experiment number 1 with the second experiment. In doing so, it is common for the experimenter to conclude that it is better to change the OFD or SID. Such a conclusion is invalid. The concept of magnification is a result of the OFD and SOD ratio. Thus, the conclusion should address this concept. As a result, the actual conclusion for this experiment is that the best radiographic quality is obtained with a small OFD to SOD ratio (OFD is small and SOD is large).

ANSWERS TO QUESTIONS

1. Define magnification.

In magnification, the size of the object increases, but the shape of the object remains unchanged.

2. What is the relationship of the OFD to SOD ratio if a large amount of blurring is visible on the radiograph?

The OFD to SOD ratio is large.

3. What is the percent magnification if an object's size is 15 cm and the image size is 30 cm (show math)?

$$\frac{30 - 15}{15} \times 100 = 15/15 \times 100 = 1 \times 100 = 100\%$$

4. It is important to obtain an image which has fine detail. However, a 5 inch OFD exists. What may be done to reduce the magnification?

Magnification may be reduced by increasing the SID which would decrease the OFD to SOD ratio.

44

EFFECT OF MOTION ON RADIOGRAPHIC QUALITY

EQUIPMENT

A cardboard or extremity cassette with high resolution ability is needed for this laboratory. This helps decrease the influence of external factors which may influence the results on the geometric image quality.

PROCEDURE

There is no commercial instrument available for this laboratory. Thus, the radiopaque string must be made. It is easiest to mount an old steel guitar string on a wooden board. The string should provide the capability to continue in motion during the exposure. Also, the string should continue moving until the individual who "strummed" the string to put it in motion is out of the radiation area.

The exposure should be long enough to demonstrate the motion. Too short an exposure can "stop" the motion.

VISUAL OBSERVATION

The image on the first exposure is sharp and the borders are well defined. The image on the second exposure is blurred.

CONCLUSION

Motion decreases geometric image quality.

ANSWERS TO QUESTIONS

1. What effect does motion have on geometric image quality?

   Motion decreases geometric image quality.

2. List 2 ways in which a part may be immobilized.

   Two methods used to immobilize a part are having the patient hold his/her breath and use of sandbags.

3. Identify when motion may be desirable.

   Sometimes it is desirable to use motion to visualize anatomical parts which are normally superimposed upon the part of interest. In this instance, the motion blurs the objects obscuring the desired part, thus, making the part visible.

45

INVERSE

SQUARE LAW

EQUIPMENT

There are many kinds of radiation detectors. Some are more sensitive than others. Also, the radiation output of the x-ray machine varies relative to the type of equipment. Therefore, it is important to match the radiation detector to the output of the x-ray machine. The detector should be able to accurately record the radiation output. If a dosimeter pencil is used for the laboratory, a 200 mR dosimeter is recommended for a single phase full rectified x-ray unit.

PROCEDURE

Since radiation is inversely proportional to the square of the distance, it is important that the 20 SID radiation reading be high enough to enable the detector to measure the radiation when the SID is increased to 40 inches. If little to no radiation is detected at 40 SID, the initial technique should be increased and the experiment repeated.

Radiation detectors are not 100% accurate. Also, the radiation intensity may vary for a given technique. Consequently, to reduce errors, an average of 3 exposures is made for each SID.

CONCLUSION

Theoretically, the radiation intensity at 40 SID should be 1/4 that of 20 SID (inversely proportional). However, it is rare that the radiation readings demonstrate numbers which are exactly 1/4.

To improve the accuracy, the instructor may wish to have the experimenter plot the radiation readings on log-log paper (intensity is a log function). If so, the researcher should take several intermediate readings as the more points plotted, the more accurate the results (the "y" axis of the graph is the mR reading and the "x" axis represents the SID). Once the readings are plotted, the researcher should extrapolate the results (see the appendix on Graphing). The graph should be a straight line demonstrating the inverse square relationship.

ANSWERS TO QUESTIONS

1. Define inverse square law.

   The inverse square law states that the intensity of an x-ray beam is inversely proportional to the square of the distance from its source.

2. How may the inverse square law be used in radiography?

   The inverse square law is useful in applying radiation protection and radiographic quality.

3. What is the relationship of SID to the intensity of x-rays?

   The intensity of x-rays is inversely proportional to the square of the source image distance.

46

ADDED

FILTRATION

EQUIPMENT

This laboratory calls for the use of cardboard film holders. If cardboard film holders and nonscreen film are not available, it is recommended that high resolution intensifying screen film holders and film be used. Replacing the cardboard film holder with a cassette (intensifying screen) and/or screen film introduces a loss of definition resulting from the film emulsion and the construction and composition of the intensifying screen. Thus, the effect of filtration on contrast may be distorted.

VISUAL OBSERVATION

It is usually much easier to see the decrease in density and more difficult to visualize the effect on contrast (which decreases).

DATA

The readings of the dosimeter depend upon the technique employed and the type of x-ray equipment used. In general, dosimeter pencils do tend to be somewhat inaccurate. Also, it may be possible that the technique employed to obtain a diagnostic film of the penetrometer is not sufficient to move the hairline of the dosimeter to 3/4 scale or the hairline is off scale.

In the case of dosimeter inaccuracy, the instructor may elect to have the experimenter do 2 additional exposures of the dosimeter *without* the film located under the tube and take an average of the 3 readings. This improves the accuracy of the reading. If the instructor elects to use 1 exposure, it is suggested the instructor review the dosimeter readings to ensure they decrease as the filtration increases.

If the exposure does not move the hairline of the dosimeter 3/4 scale, the dosimeter portion of the laboratory may be performed separately from the filming. This enables the researcher to set a technique specific to the dosimeter. Again, the instructor may wish to have the researcher take the average of 3 exposures for each filtration level.

The exact density figures depend upon the radiograph. However, the instructor should view the films to make sure they are of diagnostic quality (not too light or dark).

CONCLUSION

From the data and visual observation sections, the researcher should conclude that as filtration increases, density, contrast and dose decrease. It is difficult to make any statement about the effect of filtration on beam quality as there are no data to assess beam quality, e.g., half value layer.

ANSWERS TO QUESTIONS

1. What effect did increasing filtration have on density?

   Increasing filtration decreases density (assuming all other factors remain the same).

2. Why is the addition of filtration advantageous to the patient?

   The advantage of filtration is that it increases the quality (hardness) of an x-ray beam and reduces the amount of radiation absorption by the patient.

3. What effect does increasing filtration have on x-ray beam quality?

   Increasing filtration increases the beam quality.

4. What effect does increasing filtration have on dose?

   Increasing filtration decreases dose.

5. What material is used for filtration in the diagnostic x-ray energy range?

   Aluminum is the material of choice for diagnostic x-ray units.

47

REJECT FILM
ANALYSIS

Instructors may wish to add, delete or otherwise alter the standards or guidelines listed in this laboratory for reject film analysis to accommodate the needs of their specific department.

PROCEDURE

The instructor may wish to have the researchers work in small groups or if a sufficient quantity of supplies is available, they may work individually. It is recommended that those working in a group classify radiographs by *consensus*. This helps illustrate differences of opinions that arise when categorizing radiographs.

Experimenters may obtain reject films by setting up their own collection process in the laboratory or other suitable imaging department area. Allowing researchers to collect their own reject films provides an additional learning experience regarding the establishment of a reject film analysis program. However, this added experience requires that the laboratory be done over an extended period of time (several laboratory sessions). The length of time required will vary according to the method of collection and the amount of film wasted in the area where the films are being collected. An option to having researchers collect reject films is for the instructor to provide a "stack" of reject films. If reject films are provided by the instructor, this laboratory may be performed in one 3 hour laboratory session.

The primary advantage of having the instructor establish the reject film supply is that the instructor can design the supply to comply with some guidelines and exceed others, e.g., exceed the standard percent of waste for a particular category. These "pre-determined" rejects provide the experimenter an opportunity to identify errors and make recommendations. For laboratories using an instructor's film supply, the instructor should supply the total number of films used in the department during the film collection process. This number would include reject films and all radiographs "passed" by the quality control supervisor ("passed" radiographs are radiographs filed in the patient's folder).

This laboratory contains 4 different charts to categorize the reject films. The instructors may wish to utilize their own chart or edit the ones supplied. The specific chart used has no effect on fulfilling the purpose or objectives of the laboratory.

In an effort to keep the laboratory as current as possible, the authors prefer the instructor provide the average cost of one film or the cost per specific size film. It is the authors' opinion that instructor supplied costs more accurately reflect any market fluctuation in film cost than author supplied figures. The closer the cost of film to the current market enables the experimenter to get a better perspective on the amount of money lost within a department

SUMMARY OF FINDINGS

This section contains the student's summary of the information recorded on the reject analysis chart. It is important that only the facts obtained from the analysis be recorded. Interpretation of the information is recorded in the conclusion area. For example, 10% of the films rejected were overexposed.

CONCLUSION AND RECOMMENDATIONS
BASED ON THE SUMMARY OF FINDINGS

In this section, the researchers record their interpretation of the findings relative to the guidelines and standards provided by the laboratory or instructor. For example, the percentage of films rejected for overexposure exceeded the acceptable range. They also include their recommendations to correct any problems that may be identified. Care should be taken to avoid conclusions regarding interpreting high reject rates as technologist incompetency. This is particularly important for individuals using the chart in which reject films were collected by technologists.

ANSWERS TO QUESTIONS

1. Define repeat films.

    Repeat films are films repeated due to error or equipment failure.

2. Define reject films.

    Rejected films include repeat radiographs, clear films, green films and black films.

3. List 3 advantages of a reject film analysis program.

    Reject film analysis is able to improve the efficiency of the imaging department, save thousands of dollars in waste and significantly reduce the amount of radiation absorption to the patient or technologist.

4. Provide an example of one guideline an imaging department may use for a reject film analysis.

    There are a multitude of answers for this question; some examples include:

    Quality control films are not included in analysis

    The standard acceptable total waste is 8%

    Collection of radiographs is to be done by room

    No category will have a waste greater than 5%

5. Identify 2 ways for an imaging department to collect reject film.

    Common methods include collection of films by technologist, room or department.

6. If 112 films were rejected by a radiology department at an average cost of $2.04 per film, how much money was consumed on wasted film?

$$(112 \text{ films}) \times (\$2.04) = \$228.48$$